EMBRACING THE GIFT OF HIGH SENSITIVITY

A Guide to Living Joyfully

EMBRACING THE GIFT OF HIGH SENSITIVITY

A Guide to Living Joyfully

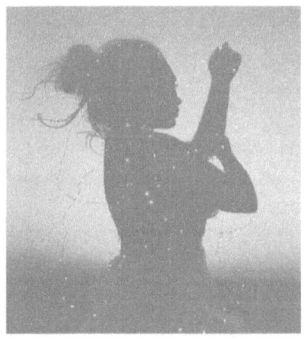

MARK WELLS

Disclaimer
The information and advice contained in this book is not intended to replace the services of a qualified health professional. Consult your physician for advice. Use of the information contained herein is beyond the control of authors and publisher, who are not responsible for any problems arising from its application.

First Printing: Brolga Publishing/Melbourne. 2021
Second Printing: HSP Health: Melbourne. 2025

Mark Wells
PO Box 79
Kew East, Victoria 3102
Australia
Telephone: 0409 985 970
Website: hsphealth.com.au

All rights reserved. No part of this publication may be reproduced, stored in a retrieval system or transmitted in any form or by any means electronic, mechanical, photocopying, recording or otherwise without prior permission from the publisher.

Copyright © Mark Wells 2021

Printed in Australia by IngramSpark Melbourne
Cover design and typeset by WorkingType Studio
Edited by Angela Rockel

ISBN: 978-1-921596-85-8 (paperback)

'Sensitivity is a wonderful and interesting thing. Sometimes highly sensitive people don't realize how gifted they are. It seems impossible to be a truly fulfilled human being, if you lack sensitivity.'

Diana White (writer)

THANKYOU

To my children, Samantha and Dean

Café Lattes

*Angela Rockel for her guidance
and impeccable 'Clean Text'*

*and my highly sensitive clients and friends,
and all other HSPs in the world for their essential
and creative contribution to the world!*

CONTENTS

Foreword	1
Introduction	5
1 How High Sensitivity Works	9
The Sensitive Nervous System	17
Emotional Intelligence	22
Sensory Thresholds	23
Sensory Processing Sensitivity (SPS)	25
Continuum of Sensory Processing	27
Sensory Sensitive and Sensory Defensive	28
Sensory Sensitives	28
Sensory Defensives	29
2 How to Recognise High Sensitivity	35
Are you a Highly Sensitive Person?	35
What We Know about HSPs	36
population statistics	36
need to conserve energy	37
are a bit backward coming forward	38
always consider their options	39
'feel' their way	41
notice the nuances	45

highly responsive	47
are easily overstimulated	47
feel emotion intensely	53
uncomfortable with change	54
remember how it feels	60
physically sensitive	62
unusually responsive to the natural world	65
concerned about the world	68
passion, meaning and spirituality	70
3 Nature and Nurture for HSPs	**73**
Nature	73
Nurture	75
Parenting a Highly Sensitive Child (HSC)	84
4 Cultural Influences on HSPs	**99**
less influenced by culture	100
Gender	102
5 Neurodiversity — HSP et al. inclusive	**115**
Disorder versus Difference	115
Recognising High Sensitivity	119
6 HSPs and Lifestyle	**143**
Balance	143
Time Out	147
Calm and Safe Space	149
Solitude	151
The Natural World	154
7 Health and Wellbeing for HSPs	**157**
Self-Care	157

Drug Use	161
HSPs and Gut Health	163
Western Medical Approaches	169
Traditional and Complementary Medical Approaches	171
Natural Medicine(s) for HSPs	173
8 Work, Career and Vocation	**177**
Which jobs suit a highly sensitive person?	177
9 Ideal Environments for HSPs	**183**
HSPs at Home	184
HSPs at Work	186
10 HSPs in Relationships	**189**
What an HSP Brings to Relationships	192
HSPs in Relationships	195
HSP in relationship with another HSP	196
HSP in relationship with non-HSP	197
11 Meditation for HSPs	**199**
Stillness Meditation (SMT) has a 'goodness of fit' with HSPs	203
Meditation for highly sensitive children and adolescents	206
12 HSPs and Spirituality	**209**
HSPs and the Search for Meaning	209
The Wounded Healer	212
Bibliography	215
Contact the Author	225

Foreword

Daily we must navigate a world full of 'busyness,' change, complexity and uncertainty. Most of us are pushed out of our comfort zones and must learn to be resilient and adaptable in the way we live, work and learn. I have spent 30 years learning, unpacking and teaching the unique influence daily environments have on human behaviour. Environments matter and they provide a daily influx of sensory stimuli that activates our behaviour, emotion, attention and thinking. We are all unique and different in our responses: what works for one person does not necessarily work for another and vice versa. If you understand how you are wired, how you respond, what is happening in your brain, what are your triggers, what works and what doesn't, life will just be easier.

This is exactly what Mark Wells brings to you as the reader in this book — a rich tapestry of insight and awareness. If highly sensitive people understand and embrace their gifts of sensitivity it allows them to celebrate their uniqueness and make the world a better place with their keen intuition, deeper thinking, and calmness. Mark weaves many elements in this book around culture, gender, age, space, environments, nature, solitude, health, wellbeing, work, careers, nature, meditation, relationship, lifestyle, selfcare (and a few more — but these were my favorites) to provide a rich understanding of the highly sensitive person's approach to life. He focuses on many elements of the highly sensitive person for you, the reader, to understand and associate, for yourself, a family member, a colleague or a friend. Through the lens of self-insight, awareness and acceptance we can learn to drop labels wrongly acquired and/or also stop judging others who are highly sensitive. Then he also brings 'Mark' and his own life experiences to the pages which provides a personal narrative that makes you want to sit down and have a coffee or glass of wine with him. You just know he will understand and support you.

The world can be a scary place and we need to be reminded that being unique is important and necessary. This is a celebration of that uniqueness as highly sensitive people.

I am not highly sensitive, actually, I am the opposite, a sensory seeker. As the seekers in the world, we salute you, the highly sensitive, and thank you for thinking and feeling more, thinking and feeling deeper and keeping our feet on the ground.

Happy reading!

Dr Annemarie Lombard
Founder|CEO of Sensory Intelligence® Consulting
Author, speaker, facilitator, coach
www.sensoryintelligence.com

Introduction

I remember the day I first heard the term 'HSP,' meaning Highly Sensitive Person, and the description that went with it. It was during a lecture and I whispered to the friend sitting next to me — 'I feel like I've finally come home!!!' It was one of those profound moments of mental clarity, similar to the moment when I first heard about Nature Cure (or Naturopathy) some 20 years earlier. The lecture, given by psychologist Dr Melissa Harte, was on Emotional Focus Therapy (EFT) and she used herself as an example when describing general HSP characteristics.

That evening I purchased Dr Elaine Aron's book, *The Highly Sensitive Person* — the definitive book on high sensitivity and how it manifests. Although my awareness of the term and my passion to learn more about HSPs (including myself) stems from that moment, my sense of recognition came with the benefit of hindsight and wisdom gained from experience — I was already familiar with high sensitivity as something I and many of my clients experienced — I had just never been able to put a name to it till then. The book explained to me in a very articulate way so much about how I experienced life. Most importantly, it also made me feel less different and less alone amongst my family, friends and colleagues! I could relate so strongly to the language used, and the way Elaine Aron described the world of a highly sensitive person. It gave me a greater sense of belonging — we all want to feel part of the team at times! I had encountered many other highly sensitive people in my practice as a naturopath/counsellor — I estimate that they have comprised more than half of my clients over the years — but in the rest of my life I was much more aware of the 'less sensitive' majority.

I have always aspired to making a positive difference in the world. Practising as a naturopath/counsellor, I have been privileged to help people achieve better health and wellbeing for 35 years. Once I recognised that so many of my clients were part of the highly sensitive group, I was able to promote and offer my services more directly to them. These are the clients with whom I feel most connected and most easily engage.

When HSPs are able to engage effectively with others, it helps us feel seen, accepted and valued. When the quality of engagement is poor, HSPs feel at a loss. One of the greatest pains for anyone in this world is to feel thwarted in our ability to contribute creatively, whether during a consultation or conversation, in the workplace or in the world. If I can assist other highly sensitive people to find ways to express themselves and have their contribution better valued by themselves and others, I am happy. One reason for writing this book is to provide another voice for highly sensitive people, to 'blow their trumpet' so to speak, and encourage the less sensitive majority to take notice and appreciate the real value of high sensitivity.

My experience and that of thousands of clients encountered in my practice over the years has enabled me to gain a deep understanding of high sensitivity. I have used this understanding to gather together information gained from research into high sensitivity, along with client reports and anecdotes, and the advice and guidance I have found most useful over the years. Anyone who reads this book, especially those who identify as highly sensitive, but also those who can recognise HSPs among those around them, will have a richer understanding of this way of being in the world. I also offer insights based on many years of experience into some approaches that support the unique needs and gifts of this group.

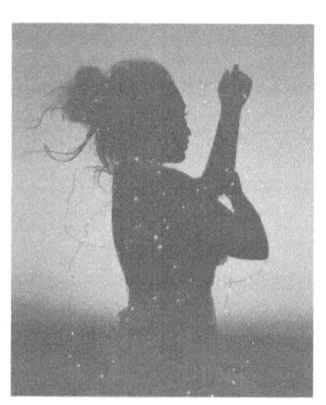

1

How High Sensitivity Works

All animals show individual differences in nervous system arousal, even when in the same situation or under the same 'threat' or stimulation. 'Within a species, the percentage that is very sensitive to stimulation is usually the same, around 15-20 percent' (Aron, 2001). The highly sensitive group has been observed in over 100 animal species thus far. This difference in arousability means that the minority group of sensitive beings notices levels of stimulation that go mostly unnoticed by the majority.

Highly sensitive animals have an obvious survival advantage, being able to recognise that there is a threat in the environment before other members of their species. However, if an animal species is to survive and thrive, the highly sensitive members must be present in balance with other 'less sensitive' individuals who are prepared to take risks — to venture out into the unknown to seek food, for instance. Two hungry wild goats might venture into new habitat that promises an abundance of food, but their survival is dependent on not falling victim to predators there. The less sensitive and more daring goat will lead the way while the more sensitive one may follow cautiously, remaining on full alert, ready to sound the alarm if they sense danger. The two goats' instinctive cooperation assures that they eat to live but also live to eat again!

When an animal species lives with cycles of varying availability of food and numbers of predators, the less sensitive type willing to take more risks by acting quickly or entering novel environments will fare better when food is scarce. However, when food is plentiful, but predators are also numerous, it works better to be more cautious about where you dine (as the more sensitive do), because even the safest spots will yield sustenance, eliminating the need to take risks or enter novel environments (Aron, 2010). During times of plenty even if these more cautious (sensitive) types feed in poorer areas to avoid conflicts, in lean years they will know better where food can always be found, having had to search harder for it.

Examples of members of animal species born with different levels of sensitivity coexisting successfully reminds me of a highly sensitive client who consulted me in my practice. He is an example of how sensitive people, given a little understanding plus ingenuity, can coexist with the less sensitive and not only survive but thrive and prosper. He repeatedly managed to create a safe space for himself that enabled him to coexist comfortably with less sensitive family members and later with work colleagues.

Michael

When Michael first came to see me about some nagging health issues he had already recognised a pattern in his personal and professional life. HSPs tend to notice what is going on around and within them, and so gain much insight about themselves and others through self-reflection. He had observed that wherever he lived or worked he would always manage to find a safe niche 'far from the madding crowd' (as he put it). Growing up with five siblings, he recalled finding it difficult and often 'overwhelming' when he was with all his brothers and sisters at one time. As a young boy it often got to the point where he would begin to overreact to everything and become disruptive as a result. As a consequence, he drew negative attention to himself and gained a reputation in the family as the one most likely to 'muck up' when playing with the others. He would then be banished to his room or sent away from the group to think about his behaviour. In time, rather than acting as a deterrent, this began to have the opposite effect because, as he said, 'I learnt to look forward to these "time-outs" when I could have some peaceful time to myself. Even the family began to notice how "chilled" I became when I had had some time to myself.' It became a way out for him when a situation became overwhelming and uncomfortable at home. Another problem for Michael was that he shared a bedroom with his 'older and louder' brother. Not sharing a bedroom was not an option because of the size of the house and the number of family members. So, he and his father (who I suspect was also a highly sensitive person) worked out a plan together. Along the back of the house was a verandah, which according to Michael, was used mainly for storage and was 'choc-a-block with stuff — it certainly didn't look very appealing. But my dad and I had a good imagination [like all highly sensitive people] and could definitely see its promise.' Michael and his father decided that they would clear it out so he could use it as his bedroom. 'I loved the idea and none of my brothers or sisters would challenge the decision because it looked so "crap," and for them was too far away from the action in the house.' This ended up working beautifully for Michael. And a few years later after a couple of his older siblings left home, he was finally able to reclaim a 'real' bedroom for himself in a now-quieter household.

It seemed that this childhood experience, as is so often the case, provided a blueprint for what happened

1 How High Sensitivity Works

throughout Michael's life. Some years later, in his professional life he found himself at a workstation that was close to an entranceway in a large open office space. He never felt comfortable with the constant traffic of people passing by and would also become exhausted by constant interruptions from fellow staff members in close proximity. He knew he was not performing to his full capacity, even though his work colleagues seemed to appreciate his presence and his ability to 'think outside the square.' He felt that he was always pacing himself and would come home feeling 'washed out' and exhausted. 'It was starting to impact not only on my mental state but also my physical health. But I'm sure only a few people close to me knew what was happening within me.' After a long weekend break from work he decided to be proactive and look for different employment, and made a pact with himself that at his next workplace he would find himself a safe niche (as he had done as a child). Within a few months, the opportunity presented itself. In his new workplace he was able to negotiate use of an office at the rear of the building well away from reception and adjoining consulting rooms, and with a view of a back garden:

> I could come to reception to greet my clients and escort them back to my office. If I wasn't seeing a

client, the office was my quiet space where I could work, away from the crowd. After meetings with other staff members I could also retreat to my 'cave.' Everyone's a winner!

His 'safe niche' enabled him to work, relax, rejuvenate and so be at his energetic best, able to think clearly and do the best job for his clients, while maintaining great working relationships with other staff.

I had a similar experience to Michael when, after lecturing for a decade at the Southern School of Natural Therapies (Melbourne), I took on a new role that required me to spend two full days per week at the institution. At that time, I had practiced as a naturopath for over a decade, consulting with clients in my clinic, where the layout catered well for my needs as an HSP. At the school, I was given a desk within an open plan office space which I shared with three other staff. They were very nice people and respected the personal space of others. Nevertheless, immediately after each full day at work there, I would feel completely drained and exhausted. The work itself was not overly taxing and, for the most part, was self-directed and drew on my creative skills, so in theory it was ideal. I persevered for a few weeks, thinking that after a while I would surely adjust to the new working conditions. But my exhaustion continued and began to impact on my other days at the clinic, and on my home-life with a young family.

I decided I needed to take action for the sake of everybody in my life, including me! I would seek out a 'niche' in the school that better suited my needs, allowing me to rest, refresh and function at my best. I knew there was a small 'hide-away' that had previously been used as a computer room and had not been reallocated. Although it was just off the main thoroughfare for students moving between classes it wasn't conspicuous and tended to merge into the background. At the same time, it was easy to find if you were looking for it — or me! It didn't have my first requirement of a window with a view of something 'green' but it was a big enough space for all my work needs and quiet and secluded enough to give me time out. It would allow me to 'come down' when I was overstimulated after giving a lecture or attending an academic meeting. When I initially made my request to move there, the principal of the school was a bit surprised, given my senior role, that I had chosen such an unassuming office space — but public recognition of that kind was way down the list of my priorities! The space worked beautifully for me and I no longer came home exhausted. I was relaxed, calm and well prepared for my lectures, meetings and other social interactions.

We all coexisted successfully. Once again, everybody's a winner!

These examples show how highly sensitive individuals who come to recognise and accept their own needs can create supportive environments for themselves. Michael's father helped him very early in life to become accepting of himself just the way he was, so they both felt comfortable about creating a unique environment — on the back verandah — that supported and worked for Michael. This in turn gave him confidence to negotiate suitable spaces in his work environment later on. In my own case, I had already established myself as a competent lecturer and knowledgeable person in the natural therapies area, so I felt fine about finding the best space — small, 'tucked away' and definitely not over-stated! — that suited my needs. In both examples the result was the ability to be productive and live in harmonious coexistence with others. Ilse Sand (2016) sums it up well when she says:

> First and foremost, you need to be able to like yourself as a highly sensitive person. And then you need to arrange your surroundings in ways that create less overstimulation for you and which are more in accordance with your needs. When these things fall into place, many other issues will

probably be resolved too, and you will feel much more comfortable, function much better and most likely feel that you have more energy for being sociable. (pg. 117)

In a fishpond there will be some fish who feed out in the centre of the pond, while others will find their food hidden in the reeds around the edge. All can coexist, live in harmony, and thereby survive and thrive.

The Sensitive Nervous System
The least developed nervous system in the animal kingdom is the Dorsal Vagal System, which first appeared in early life forms — spineless creatures that are slow moving and have few defenses. Most sensory signals come from the body to the brain (rather than being part of a more sophisticated brain-body two-way feedback circuit like that of more developed creatures). The nervous tissue of the gut is relatively large and so you could say that these early creatures' 'gut responses' are crucial for survival. These organisms 'feel' their way around rather than think their way through things. But their simpler brain still functions well in times of threat, directing the body to respond by 'freezing' and becoming immobile.

The next level of development in the nervous system of

animals is the Sympathetic Nervous System. Creatures that depend primarily on this system — bony fishes, amphibians, reptiles — have a brainstem, spinal cord and adrenal medulla. This is a much more sophisticated brain-gut nervous connection than the Dorsal Vagal system. The Sympathetic Nervous System has a developed hypothalamic, pituitary and adrenal gland (HPA) axis, which is responsible for the 'fear — fight or flight' mechanism. Motor nerve impulses that mobilise limbs, and sensation nerve impulses that send pain signals are also active. When under threat the brain engages the whole nervous system throughout the body, directing blood circulation and nerve impulses away from the gut and into the limbs, in preparation for fight or flight.

The most advanced stage in nervous system development is the Ventral Vagal System. This exists in mammals only and is primarily located in the brain and in the facial, visual and auditory muscles of social engagement, of chewing and swallowing, turning the head, vocalisation and of the heart and lungs. This system allows for regulation of breathing and heart rate, more nuanced orientation in the world, connection with others — all in all, a more finely tuned assessment of one's surroundings. This includes discernment regarding what to ignore or take notice of in relation to threats and opportunities in the environment.

With this development in higher animals (including humans) comes the capacity for *interoception* — the conscious detection and perception of sensory signals within the body and on the skin, in response to both internal (e.g. 'I'm hungry!') and external stimuli ('What's that noise?'). This is a form of perception that can be so highly developed it is sometimes referred to as the sixth sense. It is not accidental that we often use the words 'feeling' and 'emotion' interchangeably; most often, interoceptive signals are processed as sensations, but sensations are the foundation of our emotional experience, what we *feel*, even if we are not always fully conscious of them.

Some interoceptive responses are easy to identify — for example, a rapid increase in heartrate in response to a very exciting experience, and they may even take the form of highly dramatic sensations such as the sharp, crushing chest pain of heart attacks or the severe autonomic reactivity of panic attacks. But for most people, interoceptive sensations are subtle, and it may take practice and mental training to be able to consciously register these internal, body-based 'feelings.' Dr Elaine Aron and other writers often talk about HSPs' 'rich inner life.' I believe highly sensitive people have a heightened interoceptive awareness which is inseparable from their inner depth of feeling and thinking.

If we learn to evaluate our self-sensed bodily sensations/reactions consciously, we can code them as pleasant, unpleasant and neutral. These are the same categories used in Buddhism to evaluate personal 'sense-door experiences.' I consistently find that my highly sensitive clients are able to assess situations as being pleasant, unpleasant or neutral more rapidly and easily than less sensitive people.

As HSPs, if we learn to trust our interoceptive awareness it can help us make better sense of the world. Because of our sensitivity we are constantly bombarded by external stimuli that we must process and then interpret. Through trusting interoceptive awareness and using it as a guide to evaluate personal experiences as pleasant, unpleasant or neutral we can learn to better navigate the complexities of life.

For example, at a weekend party in my early twenties, I remember being and starting to feel uncomfortable to the point of nausea. I had consumed only one drink, so it was not due to alcohol! The party seemed under control, without any obvious outrageous or aggressive behaviour occurring. I didn't understand why, but felt the need to leave, so I did. I was told the next day that a fight had broken out not long after I left. It involved a number of party goers and the police were called in to restore order. At the time, I wasn't able to process why I felt the way

I did but fortunately I responded to the discomfort and removed myself! These days I use my 'gut feel' reactions to situations, people and events as a reliable guide.

Gabrielle

A highly sensitive teenage client who we will call Gabrielle had entered into her first relationship some months before. She was starting to have some doubts about her boyfriend. 'Every time we go out socially he always says things that seem unkind or hurtful. I feel very uncomfortable about it and I'm sure some of my friends do too. I don't say anything because I'm not really sure about whether what he says is appropriate or not. It just doesn't feel right though. I go home and can't stop thinking about it. Is it just me adjusting to being in a relationship? Is there something wrong with what he says? Or should I say something?'

When I asked her what conclusions she had come to after having time to think about what he had said on those 'uncomfortable-feeling' occasions she replied, 'Well, the more I think about those comments the more I realise I don't like them. I don't want to talk to or about people like that. It's unkind, it could be hurtful and sometimes what he says even sounds racist. And I definitely don't want to be like that!'

Over time as Gabrielle learnt to trust her reactions she began to intervene and tell him straight: 'That's just not good enough!' She felt better, as she was being true to her values about how human beings should treat and respect each other. Living a life that aligns with one's values, with what really matters to you, is important for everyone, but especially for highly sensitive people. Last time I spoke to Gabrielle she was still in the relationship, but her boyfriend had made some significant changes to his behaviour.

If a highly sensitive person can keep a calm and clear state of mind, they can often assess situations accurately and decide what's good or bad for them well before they are able to give any logical explanation about why they feel the way they do. I believe this is one reason why they feel very threatened when they do become overwhelmed. When their mind loses its calm and clarity they lose confidence in their gut feeling response and their ability to clearly interpret what is happening around them.

Emotional Intelligence

Individuals who are more attuned to bodily responses (or as I said, have greater interospective awareness) also tend to experience emotions with heightened intensity (Wiens, Mezzacappa and Katkin, 2000). This can work for and against highly sensitive individuals. At times, it can make them more susceptible to becoming overwhelmed by their own intense emotional responses. At other times when in a calm state of mind and not overstimulated, highly sensitive people can appreciate and use their intense emotional responses to make very discerning and perceptive assessments of their environment. They can 'read' situations with crystal clarity. This is why many highly sensitive individuals can be thought of as having high Emotional Intelligence (EQ) — the ability to be aware of, regulate, and express one's own emotions and to understand, and respond skillfully, to the emotions of others. They can be smart with their emotions.

Highly sensitive individuals naturally display strong empathy, and the term 'empath' has become a commonly used name when referring to highly sensitive people. As psychotherapist Ilse Sand (ilsesand.com) puts it: 'Sensitive people usually don't need to practice their empathic skills ... They need to practice remembering to focus on themselves.' HSPs often forget to focus on their own needs and feelings because they are so preoccupied with sensing and understanding the needs and feelings of others around them.

Sensory Thresholds

In her book, *Sensory Intelligence — Why It Matters More than IQ and EQ*, Annemarie Lombard states: 'We are born with a certain genetic predisposition to either over- or under-respond to sensations from the environment.' How much sensory input from the environment one can tolerate comfortably at any given time varies between individuals. We all seem to perform at our optimum when moderately aroused by what's happening in our environment (see diagram below). But when our arousal goes beyond this our performance begins to suffer. And some more highly sensitive people tend to reach this point of over-arousal more easily, perhaps because their baseline arousal level is slightly higher to start with. This sensory overload affects their ability to function at their best. Lombard describes these individuals as having a lower *sensory threshold*. They tend to hover in the moderate to high range of arousal (towards the right of the bell curve) unless they can self-manage and/or give themselves time out on a regular basis to come down from an over-aroused state.

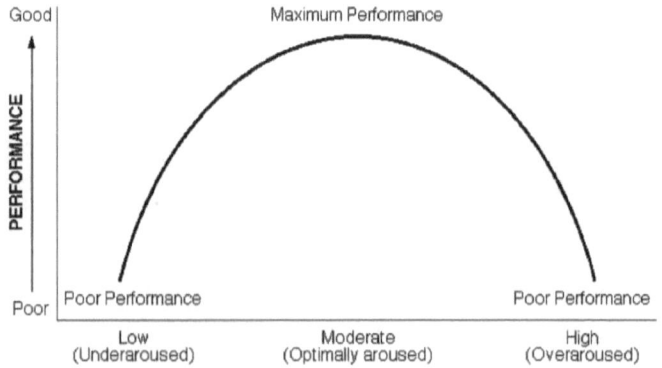

Human performance measured against level of arousal. (Lombard, 2014, pg. 115)

In her book, *Sensory Intelligence*, Annemarie Lombard (2014) speaks of a particular experience she had with her highly sensitive husband and their 2-year-old child in a crowded shopping centre. It proved to be profound for her:

> "What for me would pass without the slightest response or reaction, triggered severe discomfort and anxiety in my husband. We tend to think that everyone senses and experiences the world in exactly the same way. But our senses are unique and make each of us different in the way we experience normal day-to-day input from our surroundings. Learning to see the world through the eyes of my sensory sensitive husband has been an interesting and enriching journey. It has helped me look at life differently, encouraging me to make a bigger effort to notice small details, and to stop judging others. A few years back our shopping-centre experience would probably have left me feeling merely irritated by his 'irrational' response. Now I know better." (pg. 9)

Sensory Processing Sensitivity (SPS)

Some people love activity and the hustle and bustle of people or loud music blaring in the background. Others who experience Sensory Processing Sensitivity (the technical name for how a highly sensitive person processes sensation) and therefore have a lower sensory threshold, would much prefer a quiet hour with a book, and would quickly feel uncomfortable in noisy places with people constantly moving about. Some cope well in an open plan office, others find it distracting, energy-sapping and overwhelming and prefer the quiet of being behind a closed door. Some people are more sensitive to specific sensations than others. There are people with extreme sensitivity to being around others who are chewing food. Others are extremely sensitive to smells and refuse to stay long in some public places because of that. Others are sensitive to certain textures and this determines what kinds of clothes they choose to wear. The mother of one of my clients became frantic most mornings as she tried to get her daughter (plus two other young siblings) off to school on time. She described her highly sensitive daughter's behaviour in this way:

> "Every school morning without fail, Jenny (aged 7) changes her clothes or underwear countless times as she tries to find the right combination that doesn't itch, tickle, cut, hurt, scratch, 'electric shock,' burn, annoy, freeze or make her feel sad. I am at my wit's end. She seems to be sensitive to everything on this earth! And especially in the mornings."

Fortunately, I was able to work with Jenny and her mum to improve the situation. I prescribed some natural remedies to help and support Jenny with her high sensitivity while counselling them both (especially Mum) so that they could understand fully what it is to be a highly sensitive child (HSC).

There is a continuum that exists between those with a low sensory threshold and those with a high sensory threshold, between those who experience SPS and those who don't, between those with high sensitivity and those with low sensitivity — this is just *human diversity*. We will discuss this further under the heading of *neurodiversity*.

Continuum of Sensory Processing

<-->

Low sensory threshold   <- Mid ->   High sensory threshold

High Sensitivity   **Low Sensitivity**
Sensory sensitives/defensives   *Sensation Seekers*

Annemarie Lombard (2014) explains that a 'low threshold or low tolerance results in the brain over-reacting or over-responding ... Basic sensations have the potential to put the brain into "high alert," which coincides with a stress response.' These people seek out less sensation-rich environments, being *sensorily defensive*. At the other end of the continuum we have people with 'high thresholds who tend to under-register what goes on in their environment and can often be sensation seeking' (pg. 29).

In this book I am focusing on those whom Lombard refers to as the 'low threshold' group or technically speaking, those with sensory processing sensitivity (SPS). Elaine Aron (2010) uses the terms 'high sensitivity,' 'sensitivity' and 'sensory processing sensitivity' interchangeably. Those in this high sensitivity group face the greatest difficulties in coping with life and its stressors.

Sensory Sensitive and Sensory Defensive

Lombard divides the low threshold group with SPS into two categories: *sensory sensitives* and *sensory defensives/ avoiders*.

Sensory Sensitives

Sensory sensitive HSPs are more *passive* in their responses. For example, they are very easily distracted and affected by environmental stimuli. While displaying a high level of awareness they are likely to quickly become irritated by stimulation and experience more discomfort. Sensory sensitive individuals:
1. need to reduce the intensity and amount of stimuli
2. need to soften the stimuli and slow the pace of activity

3. need less information, and information that is more specific, to avoid overwhelm

Sensory Defensives

The sensory defensive or sensory avoidant HSP displays more *active* responses to their environment. They just as easily become overwhelmed and bothered by stimuli as the sensory sensitive individual, but they are likely to be more proactive in changing, reducing or avoiding the stimuli around them. They may establish rituals and routines in order to increase the predictability of their life, avoiding 'surprises' or novelties that may prove to be overwhelming.

In addition to the conditions listed above for sensory sensitives, sensory defensive/avoiders:

- need quiet and/or formal surroundings
- need PERSONAL SPACE
- need 'structure and predictability, sameness and routine' (Lombard, 2007)

At my children's basketball matches I found a good place to study the difference in behaviour between sensory sensitive and sensory avoidant responses to the same conditions. Any parent who has travelled around to basketball stadiums with their kids will vouch for the fact that they become either the coldest or hottest places on earth depending on the season. At any given game, you can usually see players from each team temporarily sitting out game time on the bench. On cold days I always found it fascinating to watch the different ways players on the bench would cope with the cold. Some would just sit, shiver and wrap themselves up in their jacket (sensory sensitive approach). Others would stand up, move, shake, jump up and down, and do anything to keep warm (sensory avoiders). One response was more passive (but not necessarily less effective) while the other was more active. In my sporting days many years ago I definitely took a proactive approach to the cold on winter days — I am a sensory avoider!

As part of my work at one time I travelled widely in Australia to conduct seminars, lectures and courses on Natural Therapies. To avoid becoming overwhelmed and utterly exhausted for days after travelling, I learnt how important it was to attend closely to my needs as a sensation avoider! 'Structure and predictability, sameness and routine' were (and remain) at the top of my list of personal needs. I would firstly mentally plan the trip to the airport (best times, best routes, best transport type etc.), days and sometimes weeks beforehand. Next, I knew what natural remedies I would need to take to help me avoid becoming 'vagued out' by the intense activity around me at the airport, and to avoid becoming restless, tense and frustrated while sitting in the aircraft. All details of my transport to the hotel on arrival were pre-arranged. I would also politely request that my seminar hosts put me up in a hotel as close as possible to the venue where I would be speaking. Last but not least, I would also let my hosts know that, during the seminar, I needed to be able to have lunch away from course participants and crowds. This time out to rest and process the day so far allowed me to resume teaching feeling refreshed, with a clear plan in my mind for the rest of the day. If I was unable to ensure these things, sheer willpower would get me through but there would be a big energy cost to pay the following week. Fortunately, I was usually able to convince seminar organisers to oblige me by explaining how my performance and professionalism would be enhanced by having these things in place.

Ilse Sand (2016) seems to go to similar lengths in her preparation for facilitating training days:

> 'I go over every detail in advance. I try to imagine all kind of accidents and make a plan B for how to deal with them. A more robust person ... will not be thrown so easily if things don't go according to plan. A full day of training takes up all my energy

... Therefore, it feels sensible for me to think everything through very carefully beforehand.'
Extract from Ilse's book, *Highly Sensitive People in an insensitive world* (pg. 29)

During seminars, people would often comment on how relaxed I seemed: 'Nothing seems to phase you.' Little did they know how much work had gone into being so laid back! Little did they know how many contingencies had been considered and plans of action created and firmly committed to mind. (In my own defence, when going on a holiday break, for instance, I do not prepare so methodically and do leave a few things to chance!)

Some people view HSPs as just control freaks, putting so much time and energy into creating 'structure and predictability' in their lives — but I hope I'm making a convincing case for why this might be important! HSPs' need to conserve energy is not the same as a need to control people and situations for egotistical or obsessive-compulsive reasons or because they are narcissistic power junkies. Most HSPs, especially sensory avoiders, are just doing their best to function at a level that enables them to be involved, make positive contributions, fulfil their commitments and maintain good relationships. The last thing most HSPs want is a power struggle, a conflict or negative attention, as they absorb these negative experiences like a psychic sponge. They already have enough personal challenges! And if they are in a calm head space, most HSPs will think it all through and achieve the control they need without offending or putting others out. They always consider others in their future planning because, after all, living in harmony is also in their own best interest.

Finally, although high sensitivity (or a low sensory threshold) can make you more vulnerable at times, it does NOT imply weakness! A person with high sensitivity feels more deeply, thinks more deeply and has heightened awareness and responses to a wider range of environmental stimuli than most. If we see someone walking around in bare feet and a thin cotton T-shirt on a cold winter day, we don't usually think it's 'soft' or weak for a person *more sensitive to cold* to choose to wear shoes and socks and/or a warm coat. No! We say to ourselves: 'That person in thin clothes obviously doesn't feel the cold as much as the rest of us!'

When individuals are more attuned to bodily responses they feel more, and with heightened intensity (Wiens, Mezzacappa, & Katkin, 2000). If having high sensitivity means that you feel things deeply, generally that includes pain and discomfort. But though your pain threshold may technically be lower, it doesn't necessarily mean you have less tolerance of pain. You just have a more intense awareness (experience) of the pain that must be tolerated!

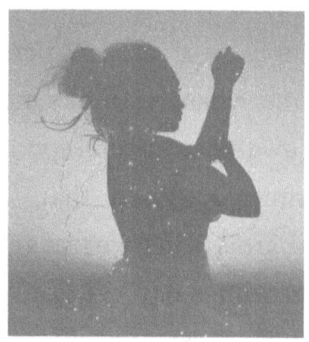

2

....

How to Recognise High Sensitivity

... excessive sensitiveness very often brings an enrichment of the personality ... Only, when difficult and unusual situations arise, the advantage frequently turns into a very great disadvantage, since calm consideration is then disturbed by untimely affects ... Nothing could be more mistaken, though, than to regard this excessive sensitiveness as in itself a pathological character component. If that were really so, we should have to rate about one quarter of humanity as pathological. (C.G. Jung, 1955 [1913], para. 398, quoted in Ilse Sand (2016) *Highly Sensitive People in an insensitive world*.)

Are you a Highly Sensitive Person?
If you want to find out whether or not you are a highly sensitive person, I recommend going to Dr Elaine Aron's website (www.hsperson.com) and doing the self-test you

will find there (http://hsperson.com/test/).

Other excellent self-tests for high sensitivity can be found on page 147 of Ilse Sand's *Highly Sensitive People in an insensitive world* (2016), or on page 40 of Annemarie Lombard's *Sensory Intelligence — why it matters more than IQ and EQ* (look under the heading of 'Low neurological threshold indicators')

What We Know about HSPs

HSP population statistics

- Biologists have observed and verified the existence of high sensitivity traits in over a hundred animal species including fruit flies, birds, fish, dogs, cats, horses and primates (all higher animals).
- High Sensitivity occurs in 20–30% of the human population. (It is a similar percentage in animal species.)
- High sensitivity is experienced by men and women in equal numbers, although upbringing and cultural influences affect its overt expression, especially in males.
- 'High sensitivity is a normal variation in innate temperament' (Aron, 2010). It is a normal trait, NOT a pathological condition.

HSPs need to conserve energy

Due to the distinctive makeup of their nervous system, Highly Sensitive Persons (HSPs) process sensory information unusually thoroughly and reflect on it deeply. If you are an HSP, you notice so much at once it is no wonder that you can become overstimulated (and at times overwhelmed) if you receive sensory information that is intense, complex, chaotic or even just new to you. Your great ability to notice things, recognise nuances and yet view everything in a larger context is also your vulnerability. With so much to process at once, when you feel overwhelmed your usual good judgement and discernment may temporarily fail you. If this happens, it is best to retreat, if you can, to a familiar and less stimulating environment and recharge ('re-boot' so to say).

I often liken an HSP's energy levels to an unplugged laptop. If the unplugged computer is left on 'maximum power' rather than 'energy saver' it will maintain all background activities and processing while also powering the work you are doing. The battery charge soon becomes depleted if it has to process both on-screen and background activities. HSPs can become depleted in the same way, just going about their daily work while at the same time doing background processing such as thinking deeply and responding emotionally to events in our lives. Unless they can plug in to the wall socket of quiet and rest in a calm environment, HSPs become vulnerable to fatigue, overwhelm and increasing anxiety. Most 'less sensitive' people, on the other hand, tend to keep the battery in their metaphorical laptop on 'energy saver' and don't process background information to the same depth while going about their everyday tasks.

HSPs are a bit backward coming forward

HSP's generally have a preference to remain in the background and feel more comfortable there. Even though 30% of HSPs are extroverts according to Dr Aron (2010), most HSP extroverts I have encountered as clients are still not comfortable being 'out front' and tire quickly if required to go there, retreating to take time out as soon as the opportunity arises. If the 70% of HSPs who are introverted are required to be centre stage (or decide to go there), you can be sure they will have checked things out thoroughly first and spent time mentally preparing. They will always display extra caution when exposed to novel situations.

My daughter and son are both sensitive. My son is perhaps closer to the middle of the sensitivity continuum than my daughter, who may have nudged her little brother in the direction of high sensitivity! They provide a great example of interactions between people of different sensitivities — and family rankings! When they were little, S. would often send D. (18 months younger) into unfamiliar situations to do reconnaissance, especially when S. was a bit unsure but still wished to test the boundaries. For example, one day when S., D. and I were visiting a new and busy playground, S. stood with D. at the entrance, where they had both received strict instructions to remain until I returned from retrieving something from the car, parked twenty metres away. S. thoroughly scanned the situation, checking out every child and every bit of play equipment as HSPs do! Her assessment was that the children's behaviour in the playground was a bit too raucous and intimidating for her to comfortably enter into yet. So, she quietly cajoled D. into entering first, just before I returned. D. didn't take much encouragement and enthusiastically ran into the playground and joined in with all the kids and activities. This way D. acted as icebreaker amongst the children so S. could 'join the party' quietly and comfortably behind him. And as a bonus, she was praised by me for following instructions and D. received a talking-to! (Fortunately, I did eventually wake up to this dynamic between my kids.)

HSPs always consider their options

HSPs need (time) to think and consider more deeply how to develop coping strategies in different situations and will quite naturally explore all possible scenarios and outcomes before acting. This behaviour partly stems from their ability to anticipate problems others don't foresee. But it is too simplistic to say that it is just because HSPs won't take risks.

My experience with less sensitive people when they are made more aware of potential problems (often by more sensitive people) is that they then also hesitate and consider the consequences of their actions. When I was in my early twenties I took part in an exercise as part of a personal development course that was designed to help participants develop trust and bond better with other members of the group. Many people will be familiar with it: you stand with your back to another participant (unaware of who it is) and slowly let yourself fall backwards into their outstretched arms, trusting that they will catch you before you hit the ground. I noticed that some participants appeared to give it no thought before falling straight back to the waiting arms of their designated 'catcher.' Others (like me) hesitated before letting themselves fall backwards. Many scenarios went through my mind in a split second. I had noticed that one of my group members was very small and petite ... *Shit — what if it's her! I'm 189 cm — how is she going to catch me?* ... Another colleague had told me he recently had surgery on his left arm! ... *Bloody hell! ... how hard is that floor?* ... I did let myself fall but the first half-second seemed to take forever and my stomach was trailing slightly behind. It was interesting that some years later I took part in the same exercise with another group of people. This time, however, the course facilitator suggested that all participants hold their position for a short period of time and consider more deeply what they were about to do. Who will be catching me — or attempting to! What if something goes wrong and the catcher misjudges? On this occasion, just about everyone felt at least a few 'butterflies' in the stomach before and during the process of falling.

HSPs 'feel' their way
HSPs are keenly aware of the moods and emotions of other people and are readily affected by them, rapidly responding to the slightest stimulus and gaining much more information than less sensitive people from non-verbal clues. Genuine empathy — understanding how someone is feeling and sharing their emotion — comes naturally to them. Dr Kyra Mesich (2001) believes a positive indication of high sensitivity is empathic ability: 'a sensitive person is empathic, and an empathic person is sensitive' (pg. 27).

All our senses provide information about our world and the people in it. We constantly offer each other visual, auditory and other clues about our emotional states through facial expressions, tone of voice, posture etc. Our brains pick up this information instantaneously and subconsciously. In one experiment researchers (Dimitroff et al, 2017) found around a fifth of volunteers — which is at least the proportion of HSPs in the general population — experienced a surge in levels of the stress hormone cortisol just watching other people undergoing a stressful experience. This is called subconscious *emotional contagion*.

Sensory clues provide information about someone else's fear or anger and a highly sensitive person will be more receptive to this information and will respond to it more deeply. Over the years, I have often heard my HSP clients say something like, 'When someone walks into the room I can nearly always tell what they are feeling and whether I want to be around them or not!' Emotional contagion is thought to be the basis on which empathy is built. Dimitroff's research found a strong link between those who are more susceptible to emotional contagion and higher scores on empathy questionnaires.

The *mirror neuron* theory suggests that neurons in the brain might be involved in feelings of empathy. A mirror neuron is one that fires when an animal acts in a certain way and when the animal observes the same action performed by another. Thus, the neuron 'mirrors' the behaviour of the other, as though the observer were itself acting. Such neurons have been directly observed in primate species.

In a research paper called 'Monkey See, Monkey Do? The role of Mirror Neurons in Human Behaviour' (2011), Arthur Glenberg stated that the brain's mirror neuron system plays a role in how we understand other people's speech, how and why we understand other people's actions and, incredibly, how and why we understand other people's minds and the intentions behind their actions. Emotions are contagious because of mirror neurons in the brain. In school I used to get a lot of laughs from fellow students by mimicking the mannerisms and behaviour of our teachers — monkey see, monkey do! Apparently I was very good at it. Although I wasn't behaving very kindly in this instance, I now understand that I was displaying a form of empathy, a trait strongly developed in HSPs, through my ability to match my teachers' moods, facial expressions, and behaviours.

HSPs need to practise remembering to focus on themselves. HSPs often forget to focus on their own needs and feelings because they are so preoccupied with sensing and understanding the needs and feelings of others in their immediate surroundings. This is a crucial point to consider when you work in the counselling and health care industry. When working with clients, HSPs need to protect themselves by maintaining boundaries, both the obvious professional ones, and others of a more subtle nature. As a colleague of mine says:

> It is essential for me to take short breaks between seeing my clients. Whether I meditate briefly or just take myself out into the garden to reflect for a few minutes, these 'time outs' are vital for me to maintain my personal wellbeing and not lose my 'sense of self.' As good as I am at understanding how my clients feel, in the past I was equally good at *taking on* what they feel as well. I not only had to learn how to maintain emotional boundaries in my personal life with friends and loved ones, but also with my clients if I was to survive and continue to work as a psychologist, which I love. I had to apply what I have learnt with even more rigor. A few of your natural remedies have been a 'godsend' too!
> Sarah (Psychologist)

Dr Judith Orloff (2018) told of how one of her clients, a highly sensitive psychiatrist, would pick up symptoms in her body from patients — headaches, nausea, back pain, depression, anger, and grief. She naturally found this overwhelming. This case takes the concept of the emotional contagion to a new level — the psychiatrist physically 'caught' what her client was experiencing.

Not all HSPs are quite this susceptible but this example nevertheless highlights the importance for an HSP of safeguarding against taking on someone else's emotions and, in some cases, even their physical pain or illness.

HSPs notice the nuances

HSPs are very aware of subtleties and small changes in their environment — not '50 shades' but '150 shades' of grey! They notice the nuances. It's as if every situation is novel in some way to an HSP because they notice even the slightest changes from what they have encountered previously. This is why travelling to new places can be problematic and overwhelming for HSPs — everything is novel! One of my highly sensitive clients, Amber, related an experience of travelling that definitely rings true with me too:

> In planning my trip to Europe I knew from past experience that I would need to stay put in places for a while to allow me time to gather myself and relax. It is only then that I can start to 'smell the roses.' For the first few days anywhere I always feel that there is so much to take in and absorb. I get overwhelmed at first then sort of go numb, unable to really appreciate my surroundings, no matter how beautiful. I need a few days to get my bearings

and once I have had some downtime to process it all I start to appreciate where I am — in time, maybe even more than others.

I had a similar experience to my client Amber when visiting beautiful Baden-Baden, a spa-town in south-western Germany's Black Forest. I had gone there to attend a Homeopathic conference. For the first few days I felt as though I was just going through the motions, thinking, 'This place is beautiful — why can't I fully appreciate it?' I would sit in the hot spa bath looking at the sprinkling of snow on the picturesque garden around me, acknowledging the exquisiteness of the situation on a 'cerebral' level, and yet feeling flat and unappreciative. The hotel I was staying at was immaculate and the architecture was lovely and still I 'felt' as though I might as well be staying in a barn! Finally, after a few more days to process everything, I began to feel comfortable and was able to relax and 'smell the roses' — just as Amber described it in relation to her trip. I appreciated my beautiful surroundings on every level. After all, as Dr Kyra Mesich (2001) states, 'Sensitive people are ... keenly aware of and affected by beauty in art, music and nature. They are the world's greatest artists and art appreciators' (pg. 21). My only problem was that by that stage it was time to leave!

HSPs are highly responsive

Boyce and Ellis (2005) describe how the more sensitive the individual is, the more 'plastic' or malleable they are, which makes them more susceptible than others to environmental influences — for better and for worse. This tendency to be more reactive to both positive and negative experiences is called *differential susceptibility*. (We will talk more about this later.) A practical take-home from this research is that highly sensitive people respond more positively to a nurturing and supportive environment, experience or intervention than less sensitive children. In other words, they respond better to positive experiences than the majority of the population. HSPs respond especially well to skilled parenting and a positive upbringing, and to skilled teaching and coaching and positive interventions in health, lifestyle and therapy. This heightened response to positive experiences as a function of one's individual genetic make-up is called *vantage sensitivity*.

HSPs are easily overstimulated

Highly sensitive people become over-aroused sooner and more easily and with less stimulation. As discussed earlier, highly sensitive individuals tend to have a lower *sensory threshold*. It doesn't take much extra stimulus to move a highly sensitive person towards high arousal.

Public speaking or just being observed critically, going to a rock concert or big sporting event is enough to send most HSPs arousal level through the roof! They become over-stimulated which then in turn undermines their ability to perform at their best.

One of my young highly sensitive clients, Bridgette, spoke of her recent experience during tutorials as a student at university:

> Every time I think of something to say in the tutorial, as I go to speak my heart suddenly beats so strongly it feels as though it is going to explode out of my chest! I am immediately struggling with my breathing as I speak, end up losing my concentration, and saying something that doesn't make any sense. There is often a pregnant pause after my comment which is bearable compared to the embarrassment felt if the tutor decides to ask me to elaborate on what I said! Fortunately, over time, I begin to feel a little more comfortable as I become more familiar with the tutorial and the participants in it. I then start to 'nail' some comments and answers. It was never that I didn't understand the material being discussed. I just tend to crap myself at the start of something new.

I can relate to this experience. A novel situation, coupled with the fact that 'all eyes are on you,' elevates most HSPs' arousal levels as it did with Bridgette. The overwhelm then makes it very difficult to function properly. Once a situation becomes more familiar and therefore less stimulating, HSPs come into their own and began to display the intelligence they possess.

Highly sensitive people react strongly to environments where there is a deliberate effort to create stimulation such as supermarkets and other shopping centres, entertainment venues, sporting events etc. I have already spoken of my dread of airports! But HSPs don't need to visit these places to become overstimulated. They tend to start with a higher level of arousal so that it doesn't take much to reach the point of overwhelm.

Some years ago I compared notes with Stephen, a colleague and fellow HSP, when we were both giving evening lectures at the Natural Therapies College. We agreed that we both found it extremely hard to 'unwind' after lecturing at any time, but it was especially difficult at night. Stephen put it this way:

> After giving my evening lecture it takes me many hours to 'come down' from it. I enjoy lecturing, especially on my favourite subjects, and get a real buzz out of it. The students are great, and they bring

out the best in me. I often find myself admiring what I just said, even as I keep talking! I don't want to give it up, but no matter what I do, I just can't unwind enough to go to sleep until the early hours of the morning. And it would be worse if I didn't have natural remedies to help me. I give myself an extra 30 mins sleep in the morning but that can cause problems with the kids' schedule etc. I love my mind but I just wish I could shut it up quicker when I don't need to use it!!!

All my life, I have had the same dilemma about engaging in stimulating activities such as lecturing or going to social events at night. When you are younger you can often recover quite quickly from sleep deprivation but it has always created challenges for me as it does for so many HSPs. Meditation (about which we will say more later) after lecturing or being out socialising always helped me 'come down' quicker from an overstimulated state. I did encourage Stephen to take it up, but it isn't always possible, especially when you have a young family and other commitments.

Highly sensitive children must learn about what overstimulates them and, more importantly, learn to recognise the signs that they are becoming overstimulated. It's complicated by the fact that stimulation often feels good at the time — a 'natural high' like the one Stephen and I both experience when lecturing. Parents of highly sensitive children, therefore, need to learn what 'winds up' their child to a point of no return and an overstimulated state that then must run its own inexorable course over the ensuing hours! With this understanding, a parent can help their child to develop better self-understanding over time. Parents can take precautions, set some boundaries, support and encourage their children to learn and practise techniques such as meditation and mindfulness. Children tend to take to meditation much more easily than adults and when they do, they equip themselves with an invaluable tool that will be of use for the rest of their lives.

A highly sensitive 7-year-old client named Bobby was brought to me by his mother. She explained:

> Bobby is a good-natured, sensitive boy most of the time but when he gets overstimulated, which can happen pretty easily, he just can't settle down for ages. I learned early to try and avoid crowded shopping centres or supermarkets when he was with me. He would so easily become overwhelmed. If he went with my husband and I, even briefly, to a crowded café or a place where loud music was playing, this would also prove problematic. It would

quickly become too much for him and one of us would have to leave our half-drunk café latte and take him outside to a quieter space. And if you added intake of sugary food to the equation, that became a recipe for disaster!

Bobby's mother had brought her son to see me as much to check him out for food intolerances or allergies (which we'll talk about later in the book) as she did to ask for advice about his reactions and behaviours. And as with many of my highly sensitive child clients, Bobby did have food sensitivities. The interesting but not surprising thing when you think about it (as this HSP author has done deeply all his life!), is that reactions to foods such as sugar or food additives varies depending on the environment in which they are consumed. If they consume the foods in a very stimulating environment such as a kid's birthday party or shopping mall food plaza, the reaction can be stronger and more intense, as it is boosted by their nervous system's response to overstimulation. At home in a quiet and familiar environment, Bobby didn't react nearly as strongly to consuming a moderate amount of what was usually a 'trigger' for him.

HSPs feel emotion intensely

Vulnerability feels like my greatest strength. It's the most human quality that allows the beauty and horror of the world to impress itself on our souls.

Frank Ostaseski

Highly sensitive people are only too aware of how their empathic nature affects them in everyday life. They too easily take on the whole world's troubles and pains if they don't protect themselves or take breaks by spending quiet time alone.

Further, HSPs often add to this distress by anxious rumination, going over and over recent experiences to scrutinise and mentally rehash what was said or done. They too easily take responsibility for situations that may have nothing to do with them, and as a result, needlessly experience distress and the exhaustion that follows.

HSPs can more easily be hurt or upset by an insult or unkind remark, and even if it is not directed at them, they 'feel' the offence taken by others. To survive socially, most HSPs become skilled at masking their responses, internalising them so that they don't attract too much attention (another thing most HSPs try to avoid).

HSPs endeavour to avoid conflict or any kind of heated discussion, as they become uncomfortable when emotions are running high between people around them. Any negativity experienced through confrontation is felt deeply, throwing them into mental and emotional overwhelm, a state not conducive to thinking clearly and contributing to a rational debate. Unfortunately, this means that most HSPs avoid the highly volatile exchanges that occur in political debate, on local councils, in many company boardrooms etc, where it seems that heated debates and verbal abuse are the norm. Until these institutions become more respectful and less combative — if human nature will ever allow it! — most HSPs will choose to make their extraordinary and invaluable contributions to society through other avenues. Luckily, as natural innovators who are surprisingly comfortable letting their imagination take their thinking 'outside the square,' HSPs will always find ways to express themselves.

HSPs are uncomfortable with change
My ex-wife, with whom I am on very good terms, has often said to me, 'You hate change — it makes your anxiety levels go through the roof. You get so overwhelmed when new information and activities and experiences need to be processed in a short time.' My reply: 'That's true, but I get through, don't I? I need a few days of time out to recover afterwards, but I do get

the job done. I don't avoid change if it's unavoidable. But yes, it always takes a big toll, and I would be happy to do without it!' My ex-wife: 'Well I have to admit you *have* often made significant changes in your life — and it backs up what you are saying.'

I have always observed that because HSPs notice so much, even familiar experiences seem slightly novel because they are aware of tiny differences with each repetition. Any major change that involves a plethora of new, unfamiliar elements to manage will be extremely challenging.

I remember a highly sensitive client, Claire, who was a teacher — a tough gig for an HSP but one they often excel at. Their ability to notice everything that is going on for each person in their classroom allows them to engage and meet individual needs. However, that asset can make them vulnerable to burnout if they don't allow for their sensitivity and take necessary precautions along the way. As Claire explained to me:

> A change of class at the start of the new school year is always both exciting and terrifying for me. The first day with a new class is especially overwhelming. So much to take in about each student in front of me. But I eventually settle into it after a few days and start to perform as I know I can. But even

then, there is no rest for the wicked. If one child is away or a new one joins the class, for instance, I am acutely aware of this. Any subtle change in the dynamic of the group keeps me hypervigilant from one day to the next. I have come to accept the old saying: 'Change is the only constant in life'!

Highly sensitive children (HSCs), experience intense distress around change. Any change — of morning routine, going on school excursions, or far worse, going on a school camp, or the unthinkable, a change of schools — can create great anxiety for the HSC.

A highly sensitive young client named Linda was brought to see me by her mother. Five-year-old Linda had been in good health and was a happy child with no major dramas in her life, until around 8 or 9 weeks before she was due to start school, at the same place where two years earlier, her older sister had begun and had adjusted well. Over the course of those two years, Linda accompanied her mother when dropping her sister off or picking her up and everyone assumed that, because Linda was so familiar with the school and its teachers and her sister's friends, she would find the transition to being a student herself easy and uneventful. In fact, Linda's parents thought she would be itching to go and excited about the prospect of joining her sister. No wonder, then, that they didn't initially make a connection between the health issues and unusual behavior she developed and her anxiety about commencing school.

The first sign of a problem was that Linda began to need to urinate more frequently. It happened when she was out, but also at home, including during the night. She even wet her bed on a few occasions — something she had never done since toilet training years earlier. Her medical doctor diagnosed a urinary tract infection and prescribed antibiotics, but they had minimal effect and the issue continued. (Linda did not at any time experience physical discomfort with her increased urination.) She also started to bite her nails for the first time and seemed to be more easily distracted than usual, to the point where she was often 'away with the fairies.'

After a time, Linda's mother began to suspect that her child might be more concerned (than first thought) about starting school despite her familiarity with the place. She decided to help Lindy become even more familiar with the school by taking her inside the grounds from time to time and occasionally making a point of encouraging her to use the school toilet. However, Linda's behavior remained the same and even intensified. She was now not only waking frequently in the night to go to the toilet but was also at times woken by night terrors.

About four weeks before school was to commence,

Linda's parents brought her to see me for a consultation. I had seen Linda and other family members before as their naturopath and counsellor and I knew Linda was a highly sensitive child but up until now she had been healthy and had responded well to natural remedies for a few head colds and the very occasional 'sore tummy.' Her high sensitivity had never become problematic because her parents understood, to a degree, what it meant and had supported her further by giving her natural remedies which I had prescribed to assist her to manage her high sensitivity.

This time I elaborated more to them on what the trait of high sensitivity meant for Linda and, with their blessing, prescribed different natural remedies appropriate for her current health issues. She responded well to these and within 48 hours her frequency of urination had normalised. On the second night after commencing the remedies she slept right through. Her other behaviours such as nail biting all but disappeared over the next week. Also, her parents observed that her general demeanour had improved and she was more attentive to what was happening around her. In other words, she was back to her old self!

A significant change to a child's home and family life occurs when he/she commences school. Even though in many respects Linda appeared to have had plenty of preparation for this event, her high sensitivity meant that potentially she might experience more difficulty adapting to such a change. HSPs notice so much that they react to even the smallest day-to-day changes in environments they are familiar with. Elaine Aron (2015) reminds us that 'sensitive children see so much in every situation, they will have some new aspects to notice even in a familiar one' (pg. 60).

Preparation and planning are essential for HSPs when confronted with changes in their lives. Start preparing well before non-HSPs do. (An early start at the school familiarisation process was essential for Lindy.) Prolong the *process* of change, but not the *commencement* of change, for as long as you can. This allows you to attend to fewer things at one time and do each one more conscientiously, often avoiding overwhelm that can arise from having to do so much in a short time frame. It also allows you to identify and address those aspects of the change that will cause most disruption. In the end, Linda was well prepared for school.

Even though Linda's parents had followed all recommendations to help their highly sensitive daughter make the transition to attending school it still remained a difficult process that required some extra assistance. They understand their daughter better now and Linda understands herself better. The change for Linda would have been a lot more traumatic had it not been for her receptive and 'open' parents who were also willing to move out of their own comfort zones to support their child.

HSPs remember how it feels

As the poet Maya Angelou expressed it, *'I've learned that people will forget what you said, people will forget what you did, but people will never forget how you made them feel.'*

HSPs generally have a strong recollection of childhood experiences. My best mate, less sensitive and with whom I have grown up (our mothers were also best friends), often questions me about my recollection of shared childhood experiences; 'How the hell can you remember that so clearly? We were only 5 at the time!' he would say, I'm going to check that out and make you accountable for what you have just said!' After all, he is an accountant by profession! Usually it must be me that brings it up again during our next coffee: 'Did you check out my recollection of that event we spoke about last time?' Sheepishly he replies, 'Ah … yeah … umm … apparently that *is* pretty well what happened.'

HSPs are renowned for their strong inner reactions, not necessarily demonstrated externally, to things that are said to them, and then bringing the issue up at the next meeting (even weeks later). Usually the other person has no recollection of what was said nor any awareness whatsoever of how it affected the highly sensitive person.

I remember a highly sensitive client who obviously had intense emotional reactions and found it difficult to forget upsets she experienced. She once said to me:

> My work colleague Peter always says things to me that catch me completely off guard. I know what he's like and yet I still get upset by things he says in passing. I'm sure he has no idea when he has offended me (or anyone else for that matter). The other day he said something to me at a work lunch; it was a remark about my new hairstyle. It may not have seemed offensive to others at the lunch but it took me weeks to get over it! That was even after a 'debriefing' immediately afterwards with a close work colleague who was also present. She displayed her usual empathy, but also added that no-one takes any notice of him anyway! Unfortunately, the damage was done. Why do these things stay with me? Why can't I shake them off? I can remember crap things he said to me years ago, word for word!

Again, an understanding and appreciation of her high sensitivity and some tools to help navigate life situations and relationships with less sensitive people helped my client. I explained that *less sensitive* friends can be educated about your needs and are usually very happy to take them into account (as you do with theirs). However, with *insensitive* people like her work colleague Peter, I hold out less hope. Maybe you just need to stay on guard (visualise a white light around yourself or do whatever works for you) when in their general vicinity and only engage with them (politely) when absolutely necessary.

HSPs are physically sensitive
I have talked before about HSPs' need to develop healthy personal boundaries on all levels — physical, emotional and dynamic. Imi Lo (2018) says 'intact energetic boundaries are needed to filter environmental stimuli' otherwise we would be constantly overstimulated. She sites Heller and La Pierre (2012, 157) as finding that environmental stimuli such as 'human contact, sounds, light, touch, allergens, smells and even electromagnetic activity' can impact on a person's compromised energetic boundaries and result in physical symptoms such as multiple allergies, migraines, chronic fatigue syndrome, irritable bowel syndrome or fibromyalgia.

My 35 years of practice as a naturopath confirm these findings. And I would add food and environmental *intolerances* to the list above as being common health issues endured by highly sensitive people (see also *Health and Wellbeing*, later in the book). Unlike many allergies, intolerances are influenced by the emotional state of the highly sensitive person at the time they are eating or at the time they are exposed to the environmental trigger. In the example given earlier, we saw how a child tolerated certain foods in the quiet of his home but reacted strongly while away from home in an environment of intense activity. And it's not uncommon for other clients to say things like: 'When I go away for a holiday or to my beach house for a break, and I really relax, eating [such and such] doesn't cause me the same problems.'

HSPs often have a strong sensitivity to stimulants such as caffeine. (I have mastered this sensitivity to caffeine and now enjoy one double-shot latte a day — a highlight in my day and, to be fair, probably my only vice!) Many HSP clients and friends are shocked to hear this about me because of their own acute sensitivity to caffeine. A long-term highly sensitive client named Christine once described in her usual colourful terms her past experiences as a coffee-drinker:

> One coffee leaves me totally strung out. Immediately, my mind races, I talk too fast, my heart beats rapidly, I become fidgety and my legs become restless, leaving me feeling 'all dressed up with nowhere to go'! If one day I developed a death wish, Mark, and

had a double shot like you, I would go into orbit and wouldn't sleep for a week! Not surprisingly, I tend to avoid coffee.

If HSPs do indulge in stimulating food or drink they tend to stick to 'just a weak coffee, no sugar' ... 'a weak tea' ... 'a green tea' ... 'half a glass of wine' ... 'two small squares of chocolate' ... if they're not me, that is!

As mentioned earlier, I see many HSPs in my practice. Instead of the normal 3 in 10 found in the general population, about 3 in 5 of my clients are HSPs. Another pattern I notice among those I see is that many experience stronger responses to clinical doses of medications, including having a greater number and more intense physiological side-effects. They often respond better to 'subclinical' doses. In many cases, this is why they seek out a naturopathic approach which tends to be less invasive and subtler than most medical approaches to health management. Homeopathy and Flower Essences — a minimum dose being characteristic of these therapies — play a big part in my overall approach as a Natural Therapist.

In addition to lower doses of pharmacological medication, HSPs often respond better to less than the recommended 'standard' doses of herbal and vitamin complexes. For instance, I find that low doses of Vitamin

B (5–10 mg) work best for calming my nervous system, whereas the common 50–100mg dose overstimulates me.

HSPs are unusually responsive to the natural world

Being in nature nourishes the soul.
Eckhart Tolle

Past research has shown that spending time in nature can have a restorative effect. For instance, Kuo and Sullivan (2001) found that young adults who had a view of nature had higher scores on attentional capacity and were also less likely to be aggressive, compared to people who lived in the inner city. In an experimental attempt to address the effects of exposure to nature, Berto (2005) evaluated whether or not contact with nature could restore attention after mental fatigue. Participants were given a task that required sustained attention. They were then shown images of natural or urban environments or geometrical patterns and given another sustained attention task (Berto, 2005). The results revealed that viewing nature photographs improved attention, and exposure to photographs of city settings decreased attention. These findings suggest that spending time in nature can be a powerful way to restore a person's attentional resources.

Kaplan's (1995) Attention Restoration Theory (ART) explains the cognitive benefits nature provides. ART describes how nature has the capacity to renew attention after exerting mental energy when, for example, studying intensely for exams or working long hours on a project or an assessment. Kaplan outlined that there are two attentional systems. The first attentional system is called 'directed attention' and requires prolonged focus during which distractions must be actively ignored. As a result, the individual is prone to mental fatigue. This is especially so for HSPs if there is activity/distraction occurring around them — taking in stimuli from the environment while also maintaining focus and directing attention to a specific problem can be especially taxing. Overwhelm and fatigue soon become a factor for the HSP.

The second attentional system is referred to by Kaplan as 'soft fascination' — it does not require focus and involves effortless reflection. (For me this is a good description of the practice of mindfulness or meditation.) ART proposes that soft fascination is most easily attained in natural environments, which the theory refers to as restorative environments, as these enable the directed attention system to recover from depletion. So, a natural environment is assumed to be effective in renewing our resources, because of the way it enables effortless reflection. (It's a simple and affordable way to replenish attentional resources for anybody but especially HSPs!)

Dr Claire Henderson-Wilson (2008) from Victoria's Deakin University says, 'people are linked to the natural environment emotionally, cognitively, aesthetically and even spiritually.' Being immersed in nature can restore people mentally. HSPs seem to benefit even more than others from spending time away from the human, built environment; the wider-than-human, natural world is particularly therapeutic for them. It is essential for me and many of my HSP clients to get out and commune in this way at least once a day. There is a tree-lined track within a small parkland situated between my home and my practice. Most days I stop off on my commute home after work and take a stroll there for 5 or 10 minutes — it refreshes me and helps to create and maintain a healthy boundary between my work and personal life.

Tapping into the plenitude of nature is a way of replenishing your energy, providing soul food to strengthen the boundaries of your subtle being and boosting your natural resilience and immunity. HSPs are especially receptive to the life force in nature whether in a garden, walking in a park or travelling out of the suburbs to spend time in the countryside. They are linked to the natural environment emotionally and spiritually — this is definitely one time their permeable boundaries work in their favour!

My highly sensitive clients repeatedly speak of how important it is for their state of mind to be regularly immersed in nature in some form or another. One client who we call Rosy puts it this way:

> When I was younger, I had several chemical addictions and obsessive habits. Through hard work over the years I have overcome most of them. I have maintained a few less harmful ones that are part of my daily rituals — like you Mark, I savour my one coffee a day!
>
> But I have also added several very healthy ones [habits]. One is my daily walk down by the river near me — I can't do without it, and I just don't feel the same if I miss it. If my world is closing in on me I can always rely on my walk in Nature to set me free again!

HSPs are concerned about the world

HSPs have an unusually strong concern for social issues relating to justice, the environment and human and animal suffering.

I remember as a 6-year-old playing on the beach with some friends, running along the sand to a place where we had to jump over a raw sewage outlet trailing out into the bay. This was in the early 1960s in a small, undeveloped coastal holiday town. Even though I was with other children who were some years older than me, I was the only one who expressed any concern. When I said: 'This is raw sewage and it's going straight into the bay!' they replied with distinct indifference, 'Yeah — once it goes into the bay it's gone.' Even at that age I was thinking, 'No! It doesn't just go away — it's in the bay ... what about the fishes ... what about when the bay fills up with it?' I couldn't understand why they didn't care. I was really worried about the sea and everything in it — and I still am.

HSPs do care, and they have a high degree of compassion. In grade four at the age of eight, behaving like an easily distracted, highly sensitive child, I got into trouble in class. The teacher took me aside and after giving me a thorough dressing down, said she was going to move me away from my best mate and sit me somewhere else, away from distractions. Where would I like to sit? (She was obviously in a good mood that day!) I chose to sit beside Paul, who sat alone at his desk — the only boy in the room who did so. He had been born with a severe cleft palate. This was in the 1960s, when corrective surgery was not nearly as advanced as it is today and so it remained very obvious. I'm sure our teacher targeted him because of the way he looked and had placed him on his own early in the year. (Her class pet was the most conventionally 'good-looking' student in the group.)

Kids can be cruel, especially when a shallow person such as this teacher sets the example. It had worried me all year and I felt extremely sorry for him — here was an opportunity to help make him feel at least a little less alienated. The teacher looked at me with surprise: 'Do you really want to sit beside ... *him*?' I made the move to his desk and we became good friends.

All HSPs are very sensitive to their immediate environment and the people in it — and they are also very aware of the impact they have on their environment. If a person is very sensitive to what others do to them but not so sensitive about what they are doing to others, I would question whether they have the trait of high sensitivity, because strong empathy is such an integral part of being an HSP.

HSPs and passion, meaning and spirituality
Highly sensitive people are often drawn to the arts and are also very artistic themselves, especially when brought up in an environment that supports their artistic expression. It goes without saying that someone who feels deeply will also be passionate about subjects that are meaningful to them. The arts provide an HSP

with the opportunity and platform to express some of their deeper and more passion-filled responses to life and existence. They present these responses in a form that demands of the observer, the reader or the enquirer the kind of contemplation that produced the creative work itself. When work of this kind gains the attention of the less sensitive majority, the HSP can feel truly heard, and believe for that moment as though we are all on the same wavelength. Feeling heard in this way is a unifying experience, somewhat like the effects of meditation, bringing a sense of oneness and a sense that we are all in this together. There is more on this subject in the Meditation chapter.

HSPs naturally and easily fall into deep contemplation, whether reflecting on the meaning of life or on how they are going to navigate the busy shopping centre to get their groceries today (and as an HSP they could easily find themselves contemplating both at the same time)! As I have mentioned many times already, an HSP must find meaning and a sense of purpose in their work, their relationships and their existence if they are to survive and reach some inner contentment. These deep thinking and feeling responses to life can be thought of as a form of spirituality and most HSPs develop some type of spiritual aspiration, whether it takes the form of religious affiliation, a philosophy, or simply a heightened awareness of their own being as a temple of the spirit. Questions about life come from so deep within the HSP's psyche that their processes of thought and reflection feel to them like prayer or conversation with their God. These experiences are discussed further in the chapter on Spirituality.

3

Nature and Nurture for HSPs

Nature

We are born with a certain genetic predisposition to either over- or under-respond to sensations from the environment ... you are born with your threshold.

(Lombard, 2014 pg. 28)

Psychologist Jeremy Kogan conducted research on 500 four-month-old babies and found that about one in five babies reacted to stimuli differently compared with the majority. In his book *The Long Shadow of Temperament* (2004) he refers to this significant minority as being 'highly reactive' — a term that Dr Elaine Aron and Jeremy Kogan believe is interchangeable with 'highly sensitive.' Kogan notes that these babies were more vigilant and cautious than the majority. They consistently register a higher degree of arousal when subjected to different environmental stimuli such as bursting balloons, unfamiliar coloured mobiles, their mother smiling at them etc.

Kogan's team (2004) found that these children had greater brain wave activity in the right prefrontal cortex — an area behind the right forehead involved in emotional regulation, impulse control, and planning. They also found that the children's skin was cooler over the right forehead, and their right inner ear was warmer than the left. This was indicative of more blood flowing into the right prefrontal cortex to provide oxygen for the ramped-up neurons there that were working hard to regulate strong emotional reactions.

These same highly reactive children had follow-ups at 2, 4, 7 and 11 years of age and in every case, as they grew older, they continued to stand out by reacting more strongly to similar inputs and new environmental stimuli appropriate to their age.

From my experience with highly sensitive clients, being 'highly reactive' does not necessarily mean that they are overtly and demonstrably reactive. Ilse Sand (2016) reminds us that despite being more demonstrative (crying, waving etc.) as infants, highly sensitive people 'are likely to grow up to be quiet and more reserved youngsters.' Their strong reactions register internally.

Nurture

Our upbringing is based on our environment, culture and role models ... Thresholds are moulded through the way we are brought up.

(Lombard 2014, pg. 28)

During my many years in practice I have very rarely encountered a highly sensitive child who does not have at least one parent who is also an HSP. The research of Kogan et al. (2004) cited earlier supports my observation that high sensitivity traits are genetically passed from generation to generation. But nurture plays a crucial role too. Ilse Sand (2016) states that 'when it comes to sensitivity, environment and upbringing are significant in determining whether [high sensitivity] becomes a vulnerability or a resource' (pg. 134). With a positive upbringing your sensitivity to the environment can be experienced as an asset. However, according to Carl Jung (Sand, 2018), our environment during our upbringing can push people 'so that they develop into a different type than the one to which they are born genetically disposed (pg. 34). When this happens, it does so at a high cost to the individual:

As a rule, whenever such a falsification of type takes

place as a result of parental influence, the individual becomes neurotic later, and can be cured only by developing the attitude consonant with his nature.

(Jung, 1976, *Psychological Types* pg. 332)

Living in a manner that is NOT in accordance with one's true nature will inevitably become detrimental to one's mental wellbeing. The only way to heal this situation is to make the change to *being true to self*. The too-often-insensitive world today makes it a challenge for the sensitive person to live an authentic life. Nevertheless, it is paramount for their survival to at least aspire to this ideal.

Not only parents but role models outside the immediate family can significantly influence how HSPs cope with and express their inherited trait of high sensitivity. I attended an all-boys Catholic school in the 60s and 70s. The cultural expectation that 'boys don't cry' was entrenched, while corporal punishment (which was legal at that time) permitted teachers — our role models in authority — to regularly physically assault us. To add to this, most students were aware of a couple of 'suspect' teachers, who, if given any opportunity, would engage in some form of sexual abuse. Years later, one of them went to jail for his crimes. I now know that at least two students from my year were targeted, harassed and sexually abused. I was never targeted beyond having a few comments directed at me that would definitely be regarded today as attempts at 'grooming.' I was spared the ongoing, deep emotional suffering that victims endure for the rest of their lives.

For the rest of us, even the awareness that this was happening around us, and the need to remain vigilant about it, could be traumatic in itself for developing eight- and nine-year-old minds. Contemplating and trying to fathom, at such a young age, why or how such things exist can easily create a damaging, premature loss of innocence in a child. And being the classical deep-thinking, deep-feeling and acutely aware highly sensitive child that I was, I found it difficult not to think about it. This, plus the ever-present threat of physical abuse from teachers and the need to maintain my place in the 'pecking order' within an all-male school in the late '60s kept me hypervigilant and overstimulated much of the time.

It felt like an intense environment in which primal instincts had free rein — and there was certainly no place for sensitivity or tenderness. Any such display would be seen as a weakness, a sign of vulnerability, and/or that you were 'homo' (in the language of the day over 50 years ago remember!). At the very least it would be viewed as a sign that you needed to be 'toughened up' for your own good if you were going to survive and prosper in life after school. Students and teachers conspired, in overt and covert ways, to dish out 'toughening up' measures! My school experience didn't do anything to help me respect, embrace or nurture my sensitivity. Quite the opposite.

However, this same school environment did meet many of my needs as a sensory-defensive HSP — and ironically, it did so via harsh, inflexible school routines enforced through the administration of corporal punishment. For me, these ritualistic routines provided quietude and order, structure and predictability so needed and appreciated by a sensory defensive person. And once I learned to recognise the subtle nuances of my teachers' moods and behaviours — easy for me as an HSP — I could anticipate those times they would be more likely to resort to using a cane, a strap, a wooden coat hanger (that hurts, believe me!), a book, a whistle, an open hand to administer punishment and enforce their authority and power. During those times, I would remain hyper-vigilant, strictly adhering to that teacher's behavioural protocols and stroking their ego when I got the opportunity. It didn't always work, and I have scars to prove it, but it kept me out of trouble a lot of the time.

Fortunately, my home life was more accepting and supportive of my high sensitivity. My father was definitely highly sensitive, and my mother was also sensitive — though less so than my father. HSCs notice more and this makes them more aware not only of negative things in their environment but also positive things — and this definitely applies to their experience of their parents. Most parents try hard to understand their children and raise them in the best way they can. Aron (2001) believes that 'a sensitive child's realization of these good intentions can provide a stronger than usual feeling of being loved.' I hope this is a comforting thought for all those well-intentioned parents who question their own ability! Even more than life experience and practical knowledge, the most important aspect in developing good rapport with your child is simply the real desire and intention to do so.

HSCs, more than anyone else, can sense and empathise with others' good (or bad!) intent. They are extremely receptive to the good intentions of parents even when parents fail at times to articulate it clearly in words or demonstrate it by their behaviour. This also applies to teachers — including a handful of mine who I understood had the right intentions despite behaviour that was consistent with much of what occurred in that thankfully bygone era. Highly sensitive children not only more readily notice the positives in their environment but also appear to respond better than 'less sensitive' children to a positive upbringing or intervention — a phenomenon referred to as *vantage sensitivity*.

However, a more negative upbringing, lacking nurturing and support, will have a more detrimental effect on them than on less sensitive children. The potential to be more reactive to a positive upbringing while also being more reactive to a negative one is referred to as *differential susceptibility*. Jay Belsky (2005) describes a particular group that are more affected by their rearing experiences than others — both for better and for worse. Due to their biological, temperamental and/or behavioural characteristics, this more sensitive group are more vulnerable to the adverse effects of negative experiences whereas others who are less sensitive are relatively resilient with respect to them.

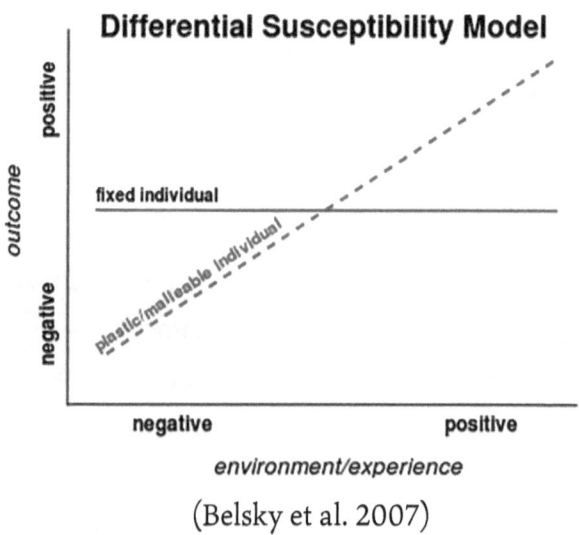

(Belsky et al. 2007)

The lines depict two groups that differ in their responsiveness to the environment: the 'plastic/malleable' (more sensitive) group is disproportionately more affected by both negative and positive environments compared to the 'fixed' (less sensitive) group.

In his book, *The Orchid and the Dandelion: Why Some Children Struggle and How All Can Thrive*(2019), Thomas Boyce describes a sensitive 'orchid' group of children as being more open, permeable, and tender to their surroundings, for good and ill. Like an orchid, if they are planted in supportive, nurturing environments, they will bloom into the most superb flowers; if they are in the wrong soil — mired in adversity — they will be more devastated than the average person. Less sensitive 'dandelion' children, on the other hand, seem 'constitutionally untethered' to their environments, which don't seem to matter as much to their ultimate development.

Boyce and Ellis (2005) described how individuals vary in the degree to which they are vulnerable to the negative effects of adverse experience and also more generally in their 'developmental plasticity.' The more sensitive the individual is, the more 'plastic' or malleable they are developmentally, which makes them more susceptible than others to environmental influences in a for-better-and-for-worse manner.

In one study, Boyce's team assessed children entering first grade, and again when they entered seventh grade. They found that teachers mattered a great deal to whether 'orchid' children fared well or not. If highly sensitive children experienced a lot of conflict with their first-grade teachers, they had 'concerningly high levels' of mental health problems by seventh grade. Orchid children who experienced little conflict with their teachers in first grade had extraordinarily *low* rates of mental health problems. However, the trajectories of 'dandelion' children were barely affected by the quality of their relationships with teachers.

Boyce reports that other studies show similar trends in physical health: If orchid children are in supportive, nurturing environments, they are the healthiest of all children, with the lowest rates of infections and injuries. However, if they grow up in a climate of adversity, trauma, or poverty, they are the sickest children and enter puberty earlier. This is supported by what I have experienced as a naturopathic practitioner for over thirty years, although I would add that HSCs, even if they come from a supportive and nurturing environment, may still be more vulnerable to illness in response to temporary stressors. Remember that HSCs don't miss anything — they notice everything that goes on around them! Unspoken relationship tensions between parents or ups and downs in friendship or schooling can easily impact in a detrimental way on a sensitive child's health and well-being. Again, fortunately, *vantage sensitivity* — their enhanced capacity to respond to positive interventions in the form of natural health approaches and counselling, and positive experiences in team sports and other social activities can benefit the HSC greatly.

So why has nature designed a subgroup of humans who are so sensitive to environmental conditions compared to the more impervious majority? Belsky suggests that evolution might select for some offspring who are more plastic or malleable (sensitive), and others who are more fixed (less sensitive) for species' survival — a concept we also discussed in Chapter 1. Varying sensitivities to parental approaches and environmental influences in general are explained by Boyce as a form of 'conditional adaptation.' Certain 'cues' from the environment — availability of food, prevalence of threats — trigger the expression of certain genes so that biological development is adjusted to give the best chance of surviving. For the vast majority, average adjustments will suffice. But nature preserves a population of more malleable (sensitive) humans who are more reactive. They respond more nimbly in harsh conditions and make elegant contributions in calm conditions as a way of hedging bets on human survival.

Parenting a Highly Sensitive Child (HSC)

When Rachelle Mee-Chapman's daughter was just 5 years old, she'd walk into a restaurant and say 'Mommy, why is that couple fighting?' The people weren't visibly arguing at the time. But by the end of their meal, they were. Whether she was picking up on non-verbal cues or some energetic exchange, Mee-Chapman's daughter was internalizing more information than the average person. Which is precisely what highly sensitive people do. They notice details the rest of the population doesn't. 'We experience the emotional nuances of others, and we are more aware of our own emotional states,' said Mee-Chapman, also an HSP and an author and educator who helps people create right-fit spiritual practices for themselves and their families. (Margarita Tartakovsky, 2017)

Most people are neither great nor terrible as parents — they are 'good enough.' And one child may thrive under a particular parent's care because there's a 'good fit' between them while another child may not do quite as well. For example, a less sensitive parent may not do as well with a highly sensitive child and vice-versa. However, as Elaine Aron (2015) says, 'there is always a good fit when parents accept their children for who they are, then adapt their methods to suit the child. Studies in which parents are trained to understand their child's temperament consistently find that the children of these parents have far fewer problems.'

Clearly though, in some situations trying to understand our child's temperament can provide big parenting challenges. They require us to dig deeper. *Parental mentalising* or Parental Reflective Functioning (Camoirano, 2017) is the capacity to seek to understand our own and our child's behaviours from the perspective of underlying mental states, such as thoughts, feelings, and needs. This can help us get to the heart of the trickiest parenting issues. Practising mentalising implies that parents have accepted their child for who they are (highly sensitive in this case) and are attempting to understand the child better and are willing to adapt their methods to suit their child. Parents who mentalise can perceive the less obvious and less immediately apparent causes of their children's behaviours. Mentalising involves a few simple steps:

1. REFLECT on your own emotions ** — when you are feeling stressed, for instance, pause and think about how you are feeling or thinking, and what the impact of that might be on your child. The sense

of urgency or pressure you may be feeling may be spilling over into your interactions with your child. It may cause you to speak more sternly, for instance. Engaging in mindfulness in the moment (made easier through a regular practice at other times of the day as discussed in the Meditation chapter) will help you avoid negative emotional responses.

2. PAUSE to consider your child's thoughts and feelings. You may not be able to directly observe the deep processing that is going on inside the mind of a quiet HSC. Human emotions are always layered but they are multi-layered and deep with HSCs! Your child may display one emotion while simultaneously experiencing another — for example, they may seem angry but it's possible that underneath, they are scared. I remember one interaction with my son when he was in his early teens, and as parents we were just beginning to give him more freedom and independence. He looked me straight in the eye and said aggressively, 'Dad! I've been invited to a party this weekend and I'm going!' The problem was the party involved teenagers a few years older than him and there would certainly be alcohol there. While on the surface my son's approach to me seemed angry,

I knew that underneath, he was actually a bit apprehensive about going, perhaps feeling that he might be out of his depth with the older kids at the party. I understood that he wanted a 'No' from me as a face-saving excuse he could give his older mates: 'My tight-ass dad won't let me go.' When I told him he couldn't go he accepted my answer with surprisingly little protest — which was fairly unusual for him at the time! Under his aggressive display and bravado was a layer of strong apprehension.

3. ENGAGE — as often as possible slow down and ask your child what they are feeling. Display curiosity and real interest in what is going on for them. This is best done when neither of you is under time pressure nor has competing demands on your attention. Use open questions such as 'Is there something on your mind?' or 'I really want to know if something is upsetting you.'

4. Be OPEN to new experiences — we always need to remain aware of the fact that children are continually developing and therefore changing. Something that bothered your child at one time may not bother them now.

** By reflecting on your own emotional reactions at an even deeper level, you will become more

AWARE of your own projections onto your child. Something that upset you as a child might not upset your child. And more importantly something that didn't upset you as a child may be difficult for your child to experience and may upset them easily. So always remember to ask your child how things are going before assuming you know.

By following these four guidelines children (and parents) can learn to:
- Recognise and identify the emotions they are experiencing
- Broaden their emotion vocabulary
- Be able to express their feelings and emotions
- Understand that their emotions and feelings are VALID

You may not be able to directly observe the deep processing that is going on inside the mind of a quiet HSC. But as a parent who knows your child is highly sensitive, you can at least give them the space and time to 'take it all in' without rushing or pressuring them.

In a best-parenting approach, a parent can MODEL good behaviour for their child. How we handle (or don't handle) and express (or don't express) our emotions, especially the uncomfortable ones, will provide a model for our child. For instance, if we consistently lose our temper every time we experience frustration, it's likely that our child is going to resort to that behaviour when they don't get their way. Of course we all lose the plot occasionally as parents, but we can still try to remain aware and identify ways of avoiding it happen too often. The most important thing for me as a highly sensitive parent was to use all my skills to help keep my nervous system from becoming over-stimulated and therefore most vulnerable to becoming overwhelmed in response to my children. Practising meditation daily (refer to *Meditation* chapter) was my lifesaver in this regard. Engaging in forms of self-care is essential for all parents — if we can't look after ourselves properly how can we look after others the way we want to?

Self-care as a parent isn't about being self-centred or selfish. If you're a parent, taking time away from your usual schedule is one of the best ways to boost resilience and strengthen your capacity to nurture and really BE THERE for your children. Too often parents are stressed and overwhelmed by the demands of raising children. Give yourself permission to reduce stress and be calm — in whatever ways work for you. It will help you develop a resilient mindset, enabling you to be a better parent.

Melissa Schwartz, co-founder of Leading Edge Parenting in the USA (2020) (www.leadingedgeparenting.com) reminds us that the word *discipline* is related to the word disciple or follower. We as parents want our children to follow our (best) behaviours — and they want the best from us! In best parenting, parents lead by example and take continual CARE of themselves in the process of achieving this.

As we have mentioned earlier, a strong characteristic of highly sensitive people (and animals) is their cautious approach when facing new experiences, which feel to them like an intimidating flood of unfamiliar sensations. Technically speaking, sensitive persons have a very active 'behavioural inhibition system.' Dr Aron (2015) calls this the 'pause to check system' (pg. 20) because it is designed to enable you to look at the situation you are in and see if it is like past experiences stored in your memory. Faced with an unfamiliar and novel experience (an everyday part of growing up), says Aron, '[an] HSC wants to check it out, and if forced to proceed, may protest, not enjoy it, or refuse this "pleasure" altogether ... Most HSCs seem to be poor adapters, but in reality they are being asked to adapt to too much. They are overwhelmed, or afraid of being overwhelmed, by all the new stimulation that must be processed before they can relax.' (pg. 20)

As parents of sensitive children we need to weigh up when we need to shelter them from new experiences and when we need to acknowledge that some experiences that take them out of their comfort zone must be faced and are non-negotiable for their proper personal development. The balance needs to be struck between being over-protective and allowing them — sometimes even encouraging them — to take some risks.

One of my HSP clients, Noreen, described her mother as someone who was not capable of responding to her particular emotional needs as a child and adolescent. She believes that very early in life she became resigned to the fact that her emotional needs would not be met by her mother. She learned to repress her feelings, and in doing so, denied her sensitivity, which then began to express itself through physical symptoms. She suffered from multiple food and environmental allergies, and muscular/skeletal inflammation caused her much pain as a child. Noreen said her mother was 'very attentive and efficient when it came to looking after me medically but always lacked the TLC.'

When she became a parent herself, Noreen was determined not to be like her mother and has developed a special relationship with her eldest daughter who she recognised very early to be highly sensitive like herself. She enjoys loving relationships with all her kids but is also able to accommodate each one's unique needs. And with the help and support of her partner, Noreen has also learned to accept and embrace her own sensitivity. Embracing and catering for everyone's unique needs in this way has allowed sensitivity to become an asset in the family.

Noreen's story shows that it is possible for a highly sensitive parent to simultaneously cater for their own needs (engage in self-care) and those of their children, arranging family life in ways that support each member's individual degree of sensitivity. Sensitivity in the family can become a resource rather than a liability. Ilse Sand (2017) speaks of how highly sensitive people who have not received the loving care they needed as a child (as in Noreen's case) can learn to give it to themselves in their adult life. Noreen has learnt this through providing care to her own children (this a great example of Carl Jung's 'wounded healer' — see final chapter). Remember too that HSPs display 'vantage sensitivity,' responding better to positive experiences and interventions, at any time in their lives, than less sensitive individuals.

As a parent it is important to be aware that a child's high sensitivity can also express itself on a physical level, for example through sensitivity to certain foods, environmental elements, odours, clothing etc. In my experience, this happens more frequently among less emotionally demonstrative and more behaviourally 'compliant' HSCs. From a holistic perspective, I believe these children's innate sensitivity finds its expression through physical signs and symptoms to the degree that its expression is inhibited, for whatever reason, on an emotional and mental level. Helping parents to understand and identify some causes for this and then prescribing appropriate natural therapies to assist all involved is my job as a natural therapist and counsellor.

Because each child and each parent have a unique personality, the dynamic between one child and their parent will always differ between siblings. This definitely applies between parents and highly sensitive children. As mentioned earlier, one of my children was an HSC and the other was sensitive but not to the same degree. This meant that I needed to spend a little more time engaging with my highly sensitive child, who benefitted from this. But I honestly believe that my other 'less sensitive' child did not suffer from any type of neglect — we simply had (and have) a slightly different relationship.

I have spoken often in this book about how important it is for HSPs to strike a good balance between their inner life and their outer social and interpersonal world. Highly sensitive people need balance between times of retreat into an inner world and 'out there' social interaction. Adolescent HSPs are no different but may need more support in getting the right balance and with navigating their very active inner lives. Elaine Aron (2015) speaks of how 'Many HSCs have had contemplative or mystical experiences from an early age. Even without formal religious instructions, they may have prayed, met angels, heard voices, and experienced the transcendent — and believe me, these HSCs are quite sane and normal (pg. 303). The inner emotional and mental life of all teenagers can become quite intense, like so many other aspects of their lives, fuelled by hormonal and emotional peaks and troughs that are an integral part of adolescence. But for highly sensitive teenagers, who already think and feel so deeply, it can be doubly intense! As parents we need to listen, provide space, avoid judgement and remain open-minded when a teenager talks about their experiences and ideas, no matter how deep, different and 'outside the square' they seem to us. As Elaine Aron puts it, 'However your child expresses this [inner life] aspect of [their] sensitivity, I believe it is one of the finest facets of the trait, and when it has properly matured, it is one of the most valuable contributions to the world.' If we accept and nurture this facet of our child or teenager, I believe it will go a long way to helping them find their true place and purpose in life.

I recall an HSP client saying, 'My parents used to get a shock when they heard some of the song lyrics I composed as a teenager. But to their credit they never criticised, always listened (even though uncomfortably at times) and supported whatever I came up with. I'm sure this is a big reason why today I can make a good living out of doing something I love in the music industry. Something they wouldn't have seen coming way back then!'

At the age of fourteen I read one of my poems to my mother and she responded by nearly falling off her chair! Though to her credit she never said she thought I was outright crazy, she still managed to convey the message that she found me a bit odd. (And as an HSP and therefore one of 3 in every 10 people, I guess I was the 'odd' man out more often than not!) Anyway, from then on I did feel that I needed to shelter my mother from some of my deepest thoughts and ideas. Parenting started early for me! Like other teenagers, at that age some of my life observations were confronting in their darkness, but I always felt better if I could air them. I kept writing poetry to give expression to my thoughts and ideas, even if my mother and father struggled to be good sounding boards. They supported me better in other ways.

In summary, here are some specific tips for parents that will assist and support their Highly Sensitive Child's development:

- Become familiar with your child's other qualities, not just their sensitivity. In doing so, raise their awareness of their other talents and attributes.
- Try to avoid being overprotective — find the right

balance between encouraging them to take some risks while supporting their naturally cautious approach. Your child still needs to be exposed to new experiences. (Acknowledging and working through some of your own anxieties as a parent will also help.)

- If your HSC shows interest in some new topic or experience, support them in trying it even if it is a bit different and seemingly outside the norm, especially if you have no knowledge or interest in this area yourself up until now. Remember that HSCs are passionate young people, so to make it easier, just allow yourself to enjoy their enthusiasm.
- If your child is NOT developing interests, offer them possibilities beyond the normal school curriculum or standard hobbies. Try to think outside the square, preparing yourself for the possibility that they will need to 'chop and change' a bit until they find their special interests (or even vocation). Take comfort from the fact that when a highly sensitive person finds their true passion they will catch up with the crowd and go ahead in leaps and bounds!
- Learn to assert yourself for your child's sake. Role modelling appropriate and healthy self-assertiveness is crucial if they are to develop

it themselves. (This is very important, and I understand that it is also very challenging, particularly for highly sensitive parents. Keep trying and you both will benefit.)
- Try not to become guilt-ridden or apologetic about every little mistake you make in parenting your HSC. * Just recognising that your child is highly sensitive is already a sign of exceptional parenting!

* Don't beat up on yourself as a parent if you feel you have fallen short in some of the points above. If you have accepted that your child is very sensitive, and if you try your best even when it becomes difficult, your child will thrive. Take heart from the fact that your HSC NOTICES EVERYTHING you do for them, but even more importantly, always senses and responds better than others (less sensitive) to the good intent behind all that you do for them.

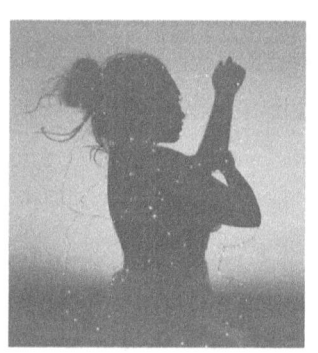

4

Cultural Influences on HSPs

Sensitivity is valued differently in different cultures and countries. Dr Aron (2001) talks of how in Japan, Sweden, and China 'sensitive' individuals command respect and are revered, and in Japanese schools, sensitive children are the most popular. She also points out that, while psychological research provides valuable insights into human nature, research 'can only reflect the biases of the culture from which it comes' (pg. 16). She points out that Japanese psychologists, for instance, expect highly sensitive individuals to perform better and they usually do. They see more flaws in the way non-sensitive people behave. Western psychological research, on the other hand, reflects its cultural bias via findings that show HSPs to be less happy and less mentally healthy — which is just not true. We could take some advice here from the growing movement that celebrates neurodiversity, recognising inherent gifts that come along with the diversity of brains.

In Western cultures, especially America, the sensitive minority do not fare so well; the more cautious 'think first,' carefully observant person is often relegated to the background by more impulsive, single-minded and self-promoting members of the less sensitive majority. 'Preferring toughness, the culture sees our trait [high sensitivity] as something difficult to live with, something to be cured' (Aron 2001, pg. 37). Later in this chapter I will speak directly to this bias when I touch on my experience playing Australian Rules Football.

Highly sensitive people are less influenced by culture

Masuda and Nisbett (2001) carried out some interesting research that made comparisons between how American and Japanese students perceive the world. Photographs were shown to students from both nationalities. After a short time had elapsed, American students tended to recall specific details while Japanese students placed these details in a wider context. Brain imaging research has revealed how cultural influences play a role in neural activation during perception, explaining some of the differences in how people in different countries perceive their world.

Building on Masuda and Nisbett's studies, Professor

of Psychology at Stony Brook University Arthur Aron and his colleagues (2010) completed another study whose findings suggests that individuals who are highly sensitive have cognitive responses that appear to be *not* influenced by culture at all. The data suggested that some categories of individuals, based on their natural [sensitivity] traits, are less influenced by their cultural context than others. 'The influence of culture on effortful perception was especially strong for those who scored low on the scale measuring sensitivity, but for those who scored high on the measure, there was no cultural difference at all.'

Dr Aron believes a reason for this may be that most non-sensitive people connect with their cultures as their reality, while highly sensitive people tend to look beyond cultural prescriptions and expectations and are open to more sources of information than less sensitive people. My experience within my practice supports this. But further, HSPs tend to be more cautious, not just blindly accepting the status quo, and think more deeply about why they would follow any social norm, especially if it makes them feel uncomfortable or overwhelmed. Most HSPs learn to trust their naturally deep mental processing to make the right choices and only succumb to peer pressure to avoid conflict. They won't genuinely conform to anything that doesn't align with their own values. In other words, my experience is that highly sensitive people want to think for themselves and have the capacity to do so! They just need to be given enough space and freedom.

HSPs recognise the fact that there are many different kinds of cultures, whereas some less sensitive people may even be willing to go to war to defend their reality, which they perceive as the only 'right' one. More sensitive people tend to see both sides of an argument so it is more difficult for them to become passionate about one side against the other! You could say that sensitive people see the conversation in the larger world — a bigger context — that culture misses. As a result, highly sensitive people by their very nature interact with the world from a different perspective.

In a testimonial to a course conducted by Maria Hill (www.sensitiveevolution.com) Tammy Junker, an HSP, wrote:

> We are all conditioned to fit in and conform. However, we are created to reform and redefine to be human. Creating is all about expressing our own unique self...

Gender

Growing up in a 'Western' culture such as Australia, everyone is influenced from birth by culture-driven gender stereotypes, through the colours used in their rooms and the colour of their clothes, the types of toys provided, the hobbies and sports they are encouraged to be involved in, and expectations about how they should behave and even the careers they should or shouldn't pursue.

Boys

Much of what I speak about in this next section is derived from my experience in growing up as a male in the 1960s, '70s and '80s. Since then, some aspects of the culture have changed for the better but many others have stayed the same.

I was involved in a lot of team sports from early childhood and I believe it had a significant role in helping me to develop good self-esteem. Being part of a team and being respected for my contribution made me feel accepted for who I was, including my sensitivity. Participating in team sports was a positive influence on shaping the person I have become. But it could easily have been very different if it wasn't for the influence of one of my early football coaches, who I know to be a highly sensitive man. He regarded himself as being 'shy' (language of the day) and perceived me to be the same. He showed empathy and understanding towards me as a thirteen-year-old boy.

Like many HSPs, I would become nervous at times in the group environment, especially when attention was focused on me, not just the whole team. When this became overwhelming for me, I would not perform to my true ability, which he had observed in quieter and less formal moments at football training. Come game day I would have already over-thought my role and all the different scenarios that could occur during the game. My anxiety levels would build over the days before the game, unlike many other members of the team, who at 12 or 13 did not give it the same deep thought and were just keen to get out there and play footy! Our coach somehow sensed my challenges and remained very patient, persevering with me despite some very average performances.

As a true HSP I was acutely aware of my shortcomings and even more aware of what other teammates might think of me if I let them down. I actually gave up after a few weeks because of it and placed playing footy in the 'too hard' basket. On the week I stopped coming to training my coach visited my parents and between them they convinced me to stay on in the team. He believed in my natural ability and said that if I hung in there I could make a good footballer. And sure enough, things did change.

There was a defining moment for me in the last practice game we had before the football season began in earnest. It occurred in the 'huddle' as it is called, when the coach gives his final address to the players before they go to play the last quarter of the game. In the first three quarters of the game I had been fairly quiet, only winning a few disposals. He decided to move me into a new position at full forward. In Australian rules football this meant I was a big focal point for other teammates to deliver the ball to. I would then hopefully kick goals for the team. During the huddle he told the other players that they must deliver the ball to me whenever possible in this final quarter. The psychological effect on me was dramatic — it gave me not only permission, but a direct order to make myself the centre of attention for other teammates. This was to be my role, and like most HSPs (apart from the occasional extroverted HSP), being the centre of attention was not something I aspired to at all.

The strategy used by this coach worked like a charm for me. He sensed the right moment to place me in the limelight (perhaps my body language signalled that I was sufficiently relaxed) and also left me no time to over-think the situation. I performed well, creating space for myself in the game and, with the help of teammates, kicked several goals, which ended up winning the match for us. My self-belief grew and I never looked back.

I often wonder what direction my life would have taken, especially with regard to sports, if that highly sensitive coach had not noticed something in me that other 'less sensitive' people did not. Most coaches at that time, especially of boys, would have just told me to 'toughen up' and would have accepted my initial withdrawal from the team — I would have been overlooked, judged as being not strong enough mentally for the game, or at worst, weak-hearted and bit of a wimp.

Dr Ted Zeff (highlysensitive.org/371/ted-zeff-on-highly-sensitive-boys-and-men/) conducted research on highly sensitive males, based on interviews with thirty men from five different countries. He found that sensitive boys who participated in team sports had higher self-esteem, and, regardless of physique, were 'never' or 'rarely' teased. However, those who reported that neither parents were supportive of their sensitivity and who never played team sports were 'usually,' or 'always' teased by other children.

However, my teammates' acceptance of my skills as a football player did not shield me from all aspects of gender stereotyping with the game. In my early twenties I copped a torrent of ridicule when I made the mistake of admitting to having emotions that lay outside the rough and tough, fighting spirit of the alpha male football culture. It happened like this: We were having the usual beer or two after a Saturday game when I asked, 'Who are we playing next week?' One of my team-mates mentioned that we are playing such and such a team, a football side who were renowned for being 'dirty' players who bent the rules as much as they could get away with. On top of that they also had a deep-seated hatred of our team. My immediate response to the news that we were to play them was to say, 'Oh shit, not that rough mob!' For daring to voice my apprehension about facing such a team (whose behaviour my most respected coach, J.J., many years later described as 'absolutely disgusting') I was subjected to a derisive and tellingly gendered verbal spray: 'You girl!' 'Gutless!' 'No balls!' 'Weak as piss!' I was ridiculed for conceding that I felt vulnerable and made to feel that I had to overcome my 'weakness.' One of the senior players even took me aside and gave me a lecture about how I could improve myself as a person, saying he was 'concerned about me' and felt I would never reach my full potential if I didn't 'toughen up.' He wanted me to display 'more heart and desire to win' as a way of overcoming my fears.

My truth, then and now, is that I *was* scared every time we played that particular team. I *did* think with dread all week about the coming game, and when we played them the thing I enjoyed most was hearing the final siren! Nevertheless, having gone back over team records out of curiosity to check my performance, I found that I was among the best 3 players from our team in 9 of the 11 games we played against them — not bad for someone 'as weak as piss!'

This fact is still lost on some of those guys to this day, while others have mellowed enough with age to admit that they too were a little nervous about playing that notorious football team. Sensitivity, like a good wine, develops with age! And even at the time, I couldn't help but notice that some of the players who were most vocal in their criticism of me, displaying the most bravado and least sensitivity, were the very ones who managed to stay on the fringe of the game and avoid bodily contact as much as possible!

My sensitivity as a young man enabled me to express my genuine fear and apprehension about my personal wellbeing but it also enabled me to make broader observations about the game and the need to make changes that would better protect all players' safety and wellbeing, especially around the long-term effects of head injuries. At the time, these views were ridiculed, seen as unmanly, and fell on deaf ears! Over 40 years later, many AFL rules and behaviours on field have changed dramatically in order to safeguard the wellbeing of players. HSPs need to be heard, not only for their own well-being but also for the benefit of the whole community. Their concerns, insights and ability to anticipate problems others don't foresee are invaluable and can certainly avoid trauma in the future.

In his book, *How to Raise a Boy: The Power of*

Connection to Build Good Men (2019), Michael Reichert describes how in America, in order to reach the cultural ideal of being a 'real man,' boys are raised to ignore their feelings or keep them bottled up. Earlier in my life, whether in the sports arena or at the all-male school I attended, any expression of vulnerability or display of sensitivity was perceived as weakness. This was and still is extremely problematic for highly sensitive males who, by their very nature, feel deeply and intensely. Reichert argues: 'Not expressing feelings prevents [boys] from understanding themselves and connecting with others in deeper ways.' He argues that we hurt boys if we don't help them value their emotions and their social connections, adding that 'the historic model of boyhood, unchanging for generations, is woefully behind the times.' Social pressures to conform are hard to ignore, but the damage they do is unmistakable.

    I and all the other boys at my school were fearful of the severe physical punishment that could be handed out at any time, but no-one risked talking about their fears. In fact, I developed a class clown persona to hide the fact that I was 'shit scared' most of the time. Other students fortunately found me amusing and it helped us all to survive. Although we dare not cry in public, we could enjoy a good old belly-laugh that was the next best thing. After all it did at least bring tears to our eyes!

Girls

Many HSPs become experts at disguising their strong feelings and reactions. Earlier, I described how not displaying one's true feelings has been expected of men in my culture. But covering up strong feelings is not confined to one gender. Elaine Aron (hsperson.com/for-highly-sensitive-teenagers-dealing-with-your-strong-feelings/) reminds us that there are families (and entire cultures) in which strong feelings, and especially certain types of feelings, are not allowed.

A highly sensitive long-time client of mine who we will call Sylvia, speaks about how her upbringing impacted on her. She reflects on how certain emotions and behaviours were discouraged and others encouraged according to gender in her family.

> As a girl growing up in a rather large family it was fine for me to become teary or over-excited and/or emotional about things ... but if I displayed any anger or aggro I was quickly put in my place for not behaving like a proper little lady, or worse, I'd get the anger thrown back at me in spades! ... my brothers, however, would often hurl abuse, sometimes even break things in a rage ... and that was just seen as boys being boys! Later in life, especially when I had young children, I found it extremely difficult

to deal with my intense emotional reactions ... my anxiety levels became unbearable ... I was totally overwhelmed for a time there and was not coping until I decided to seek help. I admit I held on to a lot of anger too, a lot of it probably justified, but I just didn't know how to deal with it.

Emotions are feedback mechanisms — feelings tell us about our current state and how we are reacting to a situation — this can then inform us about how to respond appropriately. For this reason, it is important to acknowledge, pay attention to, and allow them to be present. Suppression or denial of emotion is not dealing with emotion and it will deprive us of our ability to 'read' a situation properly and then respond appropriately. But worse, it can cause strong resentment and ultimately serious health and wellbeing issues. During Sylvia's upbringing, much of her anger became repressed. Anger, like all emotion, can be incredibly useful and self-informative. Dr Aron tells us that feelings of anger are a signal that you need to 'stand up for yourself or leave.' However, as she reminds us, it is also an emotion that HSPs often fear because by expressing 'anger you often get anger back (as Sylvia did 'in spades'!). This can be very upsetting for the non-confrontational HSP.

Other problems can also arise when expression of certain emotions is expected as part of acceptable 'womanly' or 'manly' behaviour. Sylvia's hyper-excited, or teary, sad emotions were encouraged and expected. Dr Aron (2001, pg. 82) tells us that 'unlike the boys, if they [girls] display some overarousal or emotion, they are doing what is expected of them ... The negative side of this permission ... can be that ... girls may have little practice in emotional control and feel helpless (disempowered) in the face of emotion over-arousal.' If a person feels intensely (as all HSPs do) but does not develop an ability for emotional self-regulation this will cause problems. For Sylvia, these problems surfaced when she had children, and amid the ups and downs that all new parents experience, she discovered that she had not yet learned to regulate her own emotions. At this time her ability to cope with the intensity of her feelings was pushed to its limits.

Learning effective self-regulation meant that Sylvia's emotions did not completely control her behaviour. As research at the University of Sydney into emotional intelligence shows (Davies, Stankov and Roberts, 1998), people who have this skill can actually use their emotions to empower themselves in situations that would otherwise feel overwhelming. Strong feelings are directed towards constructive activities and used to facilitate better performance — as shown for example in sporting situations when people direct and focus emotion in specific ways.

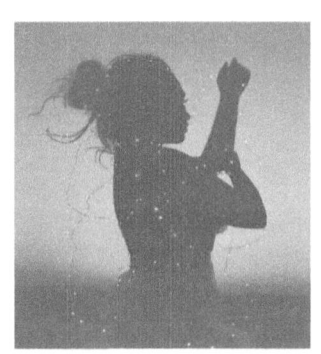

5

Neurodiversity — HSP et al. inclusive

Disorder versus Difference

> ... *maybe the bottom line is that every brain is different, and some more different than others. (Aron, 2010)*

If you are an HSP, as a child and adolescent you probably received lots of comments like 'You're too sensitive!' 'Don't be so shy!' 'What are you afraid of!' 'Don't take it to heart!' or, as my mother said to me a couple of times when she was lost for words: 'Oh Mark darling, you are a bit odd.' These are damaging comments because they are invalidating. HSPs cannot change who they are. Telling an HSP to stop being sensitive is like telling someone to stop being so tall! As an adult, when you finally start to get things together for yourself and reach a certain level of self-acceptance and self-directed behaviour you start hearing, 'Why don't you want to come out and party more?' or 'Why are you leaving so early? What's wrong with you?' or 'You spend too much time alone ... you need to get a life.'

As Elaine Aron says in *The Highly Sensitive Child* (2002), 'Trying to cure, remove, or hide a trait ... is likely to lead to more trouble. Sensitive people, especially older boys and men in our society, often feel they have to hide their sensitivity, and they do so usually at great personal cost.' Quoting Carl Jung again: 'As a rule, whenever such a falsification of type takes place as a result of parental influence, the individual becomes neurotic later, and can be cured only by developing the attitude consonant with his nature' (*Psychological Types* 332).

Variety in temperament is the spice of life, and as we discussed earlier, it is the best hope of any species' survival. Highly sensitive animals have an obvious survival advantage, being able to recognise that there is a threat in the environment before other members of their species. However, if an animal species is to survive and thrive, the highly sensitive members must be present in balance with other 'less sensitive' individuals who are prepared to take risks — to venture out into the unknown to seek food, for instance.

And if we are to survive and thrive as individuals

— no matter how different or similar we seem to each other — we need to respect and acknowledge each other's essential place and contribution. Unfortunately, the history of human beings is riddled with examples of ignorance and/or intolerance of anyone who differs from the majority in any obvious way. We often fear that which diverges from the norm and this fear can make us wary of those who are different or lead us to believe that they are lesser beings, less capable than ourselves.

A perspective that celebrates neurodiversity approaches brain differences that are not due to injury or infection as variations in human experience rather than as disorders. Jenara Nerenberg (2017) from the Aspen Institute (https://www.aspeninstitute.org/blog-posts/neurodiversity-matters-health-care/) describes a healthy approach to neurodiversity as one that

> recogniz[es] the array of human brain makeups as beautiful and natural, rather than pathologizing some as 'abnormal' versus 'normal.' It is also about recognizing the inherent gifts that come along with a diversity of brains — as history shows us, many brilliant artistic and scientific innovations emerged from those given labels such as ADHD, autistic, dyslexic, highly sensitive (HSP), etc. By embracing neurodiversity, the stigma is taken away

and we are all viewed as important, valued, and necessary components of this ecosystem we call humanity. Don't we all benefit from the passions and inspirations that come from 'out of the box' thinking of artists, scientists, and entrepreneurs? Many of those folks are neurodivergent.

I have certainly learned, like many other HSPs, that my experience of life is very different from that of other less sensitive people. I experience my high sensitivity as a gift, and certainly don't feel in any way in disorder! A disorder means someone is impaired or suffering, and my experience of HSPs is that they are not impaired or suffering simply because of having a highly sensitive brain. Likewise, many of those on the autism spectrum or diagnosed with ADHD also feel that they are wrongly viewed as having a disorder when in fact their particular brain differences can make important contributions to the world. They do not feel that they are impaired or suffering — they just feel different.

The use of labels can also have the unwanted effect of placing emphasis on symptoms rather than on their causes. When HSPs are overstimulated and overwhelmed, they may resort to all kinds of anxiety-driven behaviours in an attempt to regain some control and create an environment that feels safe to them. A diagnosis of anxiety disorder, social phobia, agoraphobia or obsessive-compulsive disorder does not acknowledge the underlying sensitivity that may have triggered the behaviour in the first place. No lasting change is possible through just treating symptoms such as anxiety, without addressing the underlying trait. High sensitivity needs to be addressed directly to improve mental health and wellbeing in the long term.

Recognising High Sensitivity

As mentioned earlier, HSPs are more prone to develop depression and anxiety if they have had troubled childhoods. But they are no more prone to these conditions than a less sensitive person if their childhoods were 'good enough' or better. 'High sensitivity is not a disorder ... only a vulnerability to a disorder' (Aron, 2010, pg. 10). We have also discussed examples of how a good and supportive upbringing (or positive intervention) will result in better outcomes for highly sensitive individuals than for their less sensitive peers. Nevertheless, the trait of high sensitivity can leave a person vulnerable to being mistakenly diagnosed as having various disorders. In addition, I have found in practice that a person's high sensitivity could also change the "look" of some disorders.

If a human condition is to be defined as a disorder it must manifest in a significant degree of dysfunction.

What's more, as Elaine Aron (2010) reminds us, 'dysfunction is in some degree in the eyes of the beholder' (pg. 199). The reactions I get when I tell someone I'm HSP can be very interesting. Less informed people — and this includes some mental health professionals! — often respond as if I've confided in them about a weakness of some sort, assuming that sensitivity must be a burden that has a negative effect on how I function in the world. Fortunately, a bit of information about the gift of high sensitivity is usually enough to change their perspective.

As discussed earlier, HSPs certainly do experience their own unique challenges in encountering difficult and unfamiliar situations, but as pioneering psychoanalyst Carl Jung puts it:

> Nothing could be more mistaken ... than to regard this excessive sensitiveness as in itself a pathological character component. If it were really so, we should have to rate one quarter of humanity as pathological.
> **(Jung 1955, quoted in Ilse Sand 2016, pg. 15)**

Let's look now at the similarities and major differences between being an HSP and a person with a commonly occurring disorder:

AUTISM

In the general understanding, those with high sensitivity are often confused with those on the autism spectrum. Although the signs of the two traits are very different there are definitely some similarities:

- Individuals with autism and HSPs can display extreme sensitivity to the environment, when it feels as if the world is 'turned up too loud,' and even seemingly minor stimuli like harsh-textured clothing or an intrusive noise, can be too much.
- Autistic children and HSPs may panic, have a tantrum, or shut down in response to overwhelming stimuli, especially if they haven't yet developed ways of self-regulating their emotions.

But autism and high sensitivity are two very different things. Bianca Acevedo (2018) of the Neuroscience Research Institute of the University of California, conducted an exhaustive analysis of 27 papers comparing high sensitivity, autism, and other conditions. Acevedo and her team found three major differences between being an HSP and being on the autism spectrum:

1. Autism comes with social challenges that HSPs do not experience. For example, people on the autism

spectrum may have difficulty making eye contact, difficulty recognising faces and responding to others' emotional cues, and difficulty reciprocating another person's overtures (think of smiling back at someone who smiles at you). These social challenges are obvious and recognised as early as two or three months of age — people on the autism spectrum 'tend to show less response in brain areas associated with empathy, social cues, and self-reflection' (Acevedo, 2018). (However, a perspective that celebrates neurodiversity and approaches brain differences as variations in human experience rather than disorders may interpret this differently. Andre Solo in *Psychology Today* (2019) suggests that 'autistic individuals have very different body language than neurotypical individuals, and they don't get to "mirror" people with their own body language nearly as much as neurotypical children. In other words, this so-called "deficit" may be much more of a lack of opportunity than an innate part of autism.'

The opposite is true for HSPs. As discussed earlier, HSPs are acutely aware of, and highly responsive to social cues such as facial expressions and other non-verbal indications of mood and intention. Also, the same areas of the brain that are less responsive among autistic individuals tend to be very active in HSPs, correlating with their high levels of empathy, social awareness, and self-reflection (Acevedo, 2018).

2. Human beings in general are wired to find social interactions rewarding — they have an inherent need for human interaction. Social bonding, helping each other out, and cooperating with one another are essential behaviours for our species' survival. My personal experience is that HSPs tend to respond more strongly to social interactions than our less sensitive peers. We are 'wired' to enjoy social situations but because of how easily we become overwhelmed, for an HSP it is always important to find the right balance between time spent socialising and time alone in a quiet environment. That way we get to appreciate the best of both worlds. For most people with autism, however, social experiences are different. As Acevedo's study points out, 'there simply isn't as much of a sense of reward, calmness, or emotion involved in socializing. An exchange with another person may get their attention, but not necessarily feel *meaningful*' (Solo, 2019). While autistic people seek meaningful experience just as eagerly as everyone else, 'the difference' as Avocedo puts it,

'is in how rewarding they find social interaction, in its own right' (Solo, 2019). HSPs on the other hand do find social interaction rewarding because, though they 'may find small talk exhausting [they] are happy to take a conversation to a deeper level' (Sand, 2016, pg. 32). As a result they tend to be selective about how they socialise, generally preferring one to one or smaller groups of people who have similar interests and life values. 70% of HSPs are introverts, and as Carl Jung pointed out, introverted people are more interested in the inner life than the outer world (1976, cited in Sand 2016) — and in my experience, this extends itself to an interest in the inner worlds of others. If I had a dollar for every 'deep and meaningful' conversation I've had in my life I'd be a very rich man!

3. Both HSPs and autistic individuals can be extremely sensitive to stimuli but their brains handle these stimuli in dramatically different ways. The highly sensitive brain, for example, shows higher-than-typical levels of activity in areas related to calmness, hormonal balance, self-control, and even self-reflective thinking. Acevedo found, however, that the brain of an autistic individual was less active when it comes to the regions related

to calmness, emotion, and sociability. Unlike the autistic individual the HSP consistently feels strong empathy and is more able to display a depth of processing through their self-reflective thinking and social awareness.

ANXIETY DISORDERS

I have never met a highly sensitive person who doesn't experience anxiety to some degree on a regular basis. It is something that I and other HSPs often come to accept and generally learn to live with. Most clients who contributed to this book have described to me episodes of pounding heart, trembling, difficulty getting their breath, dizziness, faintness, chest tightness, and fears of 'losing it' completely. They may not experience all these symptoms at once but may certainly have several in any given episode. Four or more of these symptoms occurring at the same time are sufficient for a *panic attack* diagnosis. I still experience most of these symptoms in the first few minutes of any public speaking engagement. Just the 'overwhelm' of a novel situation is enough to send my arousal levels rocketing skyward! For HSPs this understanding is crucial — that symptoms relate to overstimulation rather than social or intellectual under-confidence or under-preparedness or lack of experience. Most highly sensitive individuals feel relatively secure in themselves and are not fearful of negative evaluation, especially from those with whom they are familiar (Aron 2010, pg. 214).

For most HSPs, a key to managing their symptoms is the understanding that overstimulation generates anxiety and vice versa. This means they can sidestep the chicken-or-egg question of which comes first, and instead learn to manage both overstimulation and anxiety in order to improve their quality of life. For most sensitive individuals this will be a life-long developmental process about which this book attempts to offer some suggestions.

As a young adult, the anxiety and overwhelm from the over-stimulation associated with public speaking was just too much for me to negotiate. I got through a degree course, a 21st birthday party and best man gigs at two of my mates' weddings without making a speech. But by my mid-twenties, the internal pressure created by NOT engaging socially and intellectually became too great to ignore. Surprisingly, a regular lecturing engagement provided an ideal starting point for me. Because I was talking to the same group, at the same time, at the same venue, on the same day once a week, I quickly became familiar and comfortable in the space and time of my lecturing environment. Accordingly, my levels of stimulation declined rapidly and so too did my levels of anxiety and overwhelm. My regular meditation practice also provided a powerful tool to help reduce overstimulation.

As Elaine Aron reminds us, 'treatments [for anxiety] almost always involve reducing overstimulation first, through deep breathing, relaxation methods, meditation, yoga, and so forth.' Once I understood that my extreme anticipatory anxiety around public speaking was associated with overstimulation, I was able to take up some of these management options, developing a meditation practice and being sure to familiarise myself beforehand with the environment in which I would be speaking, making the experience less novel and more predictable and so reducing overstimulation and its accompanying anxiety. For more on this go to: *https://hsperson.com/faq/hs-or-anxiety/*

ADHD

A highly sensitive client named Steven who works as an academic once said to me:

> I know if I consulted a few psychologists I would get at least one diagnosis of ADHD. I mean, yeah, there are a few situations in which my mind races, gets ahead of itself and I can't focus well on the thing at hand. I'm sure my wife would vouch for that too! But she also knows that I have become aware of

those situations that overwhelm me. I avoid them or if that's not possible, I plan and take precautions. Most of the time my 'quick' mind works for me. When I'm lecturing, when I'm brainstorming to problem-solve or just entertaining our kids at home I'm comfortable and capable! And if I get some personal space I can easily relax and chill. Starting to practice Mindfulness a few years ago has helped heaps too.

Once again we come back to Elaine Aron's proposition that 'dysfunction is in some degree in the eye of the beholder' (2010, pg. 199). Is there a 'disorder' if someone is functioning well — or thriving as in Steven's case?

Another client I will call Jenny consulted me after she received a diagnosis of ADHD at the age of 40 and was considering using medication to manage the condition. Jenny received this diagnosis after seeking professional advice regarding an experience at her child's primary school fund-raiser. She loved preparing food and was known to be a very creative cook. Because of this, she was encouraged to work with other parents to create healthy and tasty dishes to be sold at the school fete — in a small kitchen space with three or four very chatty parents, while music blared! As she describes it:

I became totally overwhelmed, could not concentrate or think clearly. My cooking was a complete disaster! It has happened to me before on some occasions — this overwhelm and inability to concentrate. I wouldn't say it plays a big part in my life. But it is a real pain in the butt when it happens and very embarrassing!

After discussing the characteristics of high sensitivity with her, we both agreed that she ticked most of the boxes. I also counselled her about the many non-medical approaches she could take to provide a space of creative fulfillment for herself while still making room for her obvious sensitivity. Taking medication was certainly not 'off the table' but these insights empowered her to have a choice in the matter.

I too have had experiences of repeatedly losing my capacity to concentrate when I become overstimulated and anxious. From a very early age I used to spend most of my Christmas holidays staying with my best mate's family at their beach house on Melbourne's Port Philip Bay. My friend's father was a keen fisherman and would take us with him (when it was our turn and there was room in the boat — it was a family of eight children!) To be honest I'm not a great fan of fishing but went along for the ride. My friend's father felt that I had missed out on many life experiences because my father, an HSP who was more interested in reading and academic pursuits, never took me on such excursions.

When we went fishing my friend's father, with the best of intentions, focused most of his attention on me rather than on his own more experienced children. (As I begin to recount this story, over 50 years on I am already getting nervous!) Whenever you caught a fish (usually a flathead), you were supposed to haul it into the boat and remove the hook from its mouth. This was an easy procedure for others in the boat but alas not for me! It went like this: as soon as he realised I had a fish, my mate's father would stop whatever he was he doing and focus all his attention on me.

That alone, along with the accumulated trauma of multiple previous failures at this simple task (and his reactions to those failures) sent my arousal levels through the roof. I became instantly overwhelmed, anxious and unable to concentrate. The usual outcome after about three unsuccessful attempts to separate the hook from the fish was that he would come over and impatiently complete the task himself, muttering something like 'Hopeless bugger!' under his breath.

I vividly remember the last of the many trips he took me on — I have to admire his perseverance (if not his patience) with me! I knew I had caught a fish but decided, in order to avoid yet another traumatic experience, to leave it on the sea floor rather than haul it in. Unfortunately, he was on to me — no surprise given that everyone else on the boat was bringing in bucket-loads of fish. He came over, grabbed my line and immediately knew that there was something on the end. He wound the fish in and passed the line back to me to do the final honours and bring it into the boat. How generous of him! Once again I was faced with the simple, but seemingly impossible-for-me task of separating the hook from the fish.

This time I was determined to make it happen. I was 10 years old, I told myself, and stronger than last year. After my usual failed first two attempts, I said to myself 'Forget about technique, just use brute force.' And sure enough I nailed it, successfully separating the hook from the fish. However, I did it with the pent-up force of years of anxiety. As the hook hit the floor of the boat, the fish — in a very motley state after sitting on the floor of the bay for an hour or more — hit my friend's father on the side of the head and bounced. We never fished together again but my relationship with him, which hit rock bottom that day, improved from then on.

In my case, I lost concentration when became overwhelmed, highly aroused and unable to focus properly on the task at hand — even, on that final fateful day, throwing caution to the wind, very unlike an HSP. Did I display some symptoms of ADHD? Definitely. But in my case and those of the other examples given earlier, all were able to concentrate well and for long periods in a quiet and calm environment. This is not the case for most people with ADHD, who in fact often concentrate better when there is some background noise. Also, ironically, the most commonly prescribed medication for ADHD (in Australia) is Ritalin, which is a stimulant. The best 'treatment' for high sensitivity, however, is to reduce stimulation and limit other sources of arousal and stress. From this point of view, an HSP is completely different from someone with an ADHD diagnosis. Nevertheless, there is still some confusion around differential diagnoses — as mentioned, I have had some highly sensitive clients who have come to me having received an ADHD diagnosis. As always, seek appropriate professional advice whenever you have any doubts.

DEPRESSION

According to Dr Elaine Aron's research the question of whether there is a connection between being a highly sensitive person and the experience of depression can be answered: 'Yes and No' — it depends. We have spoken earlier about how an HSP is more prone to depression if they have had a difficult childhood. However, if they have had at least an OK upbringing or better they are NO more prone to depression than the rest of the population.

One important point to consider in regard to a diagnosis of depression is that most HSPs have learned to mask strong feelings, thoughts and reaction and may give the appearance of feeling better than they really do. It may be that an HSP will only share how they feel with people who have become close enough to gain their confidence, such as a family member or a therapist. The situation is further complicated by the fact that, because highly sensitive people feel things very deeply, when they actually express the depth of their feelings when in a negative state, they can come across as very dark indeed to those who don't feel so deeply. In this situation, an HSP's predicament may be interpreted as worse than it actually is. An HSP expressing profound negativity may be quite familiar with these feelings and thoughts and have developed self-management and coping skills to successfully process periodic dark emotional responses. An HSP client named Brent who has consulted me over the years once said to me:

> I always put high expectations on myself. And there is a fine line between being constructively self-critical and just being self-destructive. Fortunately

over the years whenever anything goes wrong for me, I've got better at being the constructive self-critic and engaged less in self-destructive thinking or behaviour. Earlier in my life when something went wrong for me, my parents, and then my wife in the early days of my marriage, would have to hear and be witness to some very dark thoughts and morbid behaviour. It might only last for a day or two but it certainly put a dark cloud over the household for that time. And my wife did get very concerned about my wellbeing during some of those episodes. I regret putting her through that ... I somehow always knew deep down that I would snap out of it ... I am much better now at navigating problems when I encounter them. Admittedly I don't tend to share every one of my thoughts and feelings these days. I'm sorry but it scares some people off! But that's OK. I get it out of my system in other constructive ways.'

HSPs tend to feel deeply. They experience the whole gamut of emotions from intensely positive to intensely negative reactions to life experience — sometimes in the same hour! If someone is making a judgement or critical assessment of an HSP's state of mind they need to take this 'emotional rollercoaster' pattern into account.

The most important criterion for a depression diagnosis, according to Elaine Aron (2010, pg. 204), is 'clinically significant distress' from feelings of worthlessness, emptiness, or unending sadness. This is a more useful diagnostic than the criterion of 'impairment in important areas of functioning' due to fatigue, loss of focus, anhedonia (inability to enjoy activities that normally bring you joy and pleasure) used by many medical professionals as a basis for prescribing antidepressants. Many of my highly sensitive clients have experienced fatigue and anhedonia without experiencing 'clinically significant distress.' I will use my own life experience to show how this can occur. In what follows, I am in no way suggesting or encouraging anyone to disregard the advice given by their medical doctor — rather I am offering my own experience of negotiating my path to achieving good mental and physical health outcomes.

At the age of 20, I was diagnosed with depression by a doctor who then prescribed antidepressants. I delayed filling my prescription as I was very reluctant to go down a path that committed me to taking medication indefinitely. I was hoping to work through the experience in my own way — my usual approach, for better and for worse! The significance of the diagnosis was not lost on me, and I knew I would have to be very proactive in dealing with this issue. I began to explore alternative and natural approaches to deal with my immediate sadness and anxiety symptoms, and was ultimately able to move forward with some confidence about managing any relapses.

The background of the depression diagnosis was this. I had made a decision to stop drinking alcohol every Saturday afternoon (without fail) after playing sport. I was the classic binge-drinker, starting at 5 or 6 pm and then drinking steadily until all hours of Sunday morning. This was something I very much looked forward to and each pretty much revolved around raging and partying and its associated adventures. I met fascinating people, engaged in self-exploration (very occasionally enhanced by taking certain substances) and led the promiscuous lifestyle of the seventies.

But once I stopped drinking, though I hated to admit it, partying wasn't nearly as much fun. And because of my high sensitivity — which had been somewhat numbed by alcohol — I was now feeling the full extent of my anxiety, nervous tension and overwhelm and the resulting rapid onset of fatigue. In hindsight, after giving up drinking I should have chosen far less stimulating activities and stuck to socialising with a few intimate friends before going home early! But no, I was determined to push through, continuing to stay out late and party on. I became more and more tense and anxious when I was out, and would go home so wired and wound up I would be unable to sleep. After a few weeks, this strung-out state of nervous tension and anxiety had begun to persist all week and I decided to ask my doctor for help.

I was definitely displaying 'impairment in important areas of functioning' — fatigue, loss of focus and difficulty in sustaining concentration, along with inability to enjoy activities that would normally bring me joy. I was also experiencing high levels of anxiety and nervous tension. I can certainly understand how one could come to a diagnosis of depression and prescribe medication. After all, I had already been self-medicating every week for a long time through my regular, substantial intake of alcohol!

All of this had been exacerbated by my ignorance about how to accommodate my needs as an HSP. Perhaps the most important of these, for me and all HSPs, and the one that prompted me to give up alcohol in the first place, was the need to find new direction and meaning in my life. Although this need did create a degree of discontent at the time, the 'clinically significant distress' from feelings of worthlessness, emptiness, or unending sadness were NOT present.

In the end, I chose to address my fatigue and loss of focus through better lifestyle decisions, especially around how I spent my Saturday nights! As Kelly O'Loughlin's blog (www.highlysensitiveperson.net) reminds us: 'If an HSP is aware of their sensitivity, they can plan their life in the best way to avoid overstimulation and scenarios that make them feel drained and unsettled.' I began to find more pleasure in new activities.

I also picked up a book by Dr Ainsley Meares (1970) called *Relief Without Drugs* (discussed further in the *Meditation* chapter). This looks at how learning to relax the mind deeply through meditation can eliminate the need to take many prescribed drugs. I responded well to the regular practice of meditation almost immediately and it has served me wonderfully in the long term. The whole experience also started me on a journey of exploration of traditional and natural healing methods and medicines. This not only gave me natural solutions to my physical and mental health issues but also provided a greater sense of meaning and purpose in my life — a non-negotiable for HSPs. Binge-drinking could only ever provide at best a temporary and unhealthy 'stop-gap' in this search.

I hope my case is encouraging for HSPs because it is a good example of how *vantage sensitivity* displays itself. As mentioned earlier, this is a term used to describe how positive interventions benefit the highly sensitive individual more than their less sensitive peers. Because of my high sensitivity I was more susceptible to influences that can protect against depression.

Finally, as always with any potential or diagnosed mental health issue, especially depression, a friend, loved one or therapist should always follow the fundamental principle: *cause no harm*. Make sure that your friend, loved one or client is in no danger of self-harm or of harming others. If you have any doubts, seek appropriate expert advice.

PTSD

When we hear the term PTSD, most of us think of the ongoing effects of major trauma, such as that experienced by war veterans or survivors of domestic violence. Without trivialising this kind of suffering in any way, I would like to draw attention to a related condition called *cumulative PTSD* — a build-up of the effects of minor traumas over time — which is sometimes experienced by HSPs.

I believe most highly sensitive people receive multiple minor traumas throughout their daily lives just because they generally feel everything that happens to them so intensely. An everyday experience such as a trip to a busy supermarket can have a major impact, raising anxiety levels to the point of overwhelm and leaving them exhausted! The symptoms and signs of cumulative PTSD are mostly identical to those resulting from major trauma but because there is no identifiable standout event, cumulative PTSD may not be easily recognised.

One issue that may confuse a differential diagnosis between a person suffering from PTSD and someone expressing their highly sensitive nature is the strong HSP tendency to be naturally hypervigilant. And as Elaine Aron (2010, pg. 206) reminds us, PTSD can also manifest as 'insomnia, hyper-vigilance, or an exaggerated startle response (an item on the HSP scale).' Acevedo (2018) adds some clarification by pointing out that 'PTSD patients show none of the enhanced activity in areas [of the brain] related to calmness, self-control, or social awareness that highly sensitive people show. ... Disruptions in a PTSD sufferer's brain ... tend to affect their memory and their ability to integrate new information. These abilities — and the capacity to process information in general — are actually strong points for a highly sensitive person.'

In this chapter I have only covered a few of the more commonly experienced and relatively well-known mental health conditions. My aim has been firstly to give the reader some idea of how having high sensitivity can leave a person vulnerable to being mistakenly diagnosed as having certain disorders because some of their symptoms overlap with those of high sensitivity. Secondly, I wish to show how high sensitivity can change the overall 'look' of some disorders. And lastly, I want to make it very clear that a diagnosis may not acknowledge the underlying sensitivity that has triggered certain behaviours in the first place. In this situation, no lasting change will be possible through treating symptoms resulting from the underlying trait. High sensitivity will need to be addressed directly to improve mental health and wellbeing in the long term.

Many clients over the years have made me very familiar with their experiences and have helped me to gain intimate knowledge of the mental health conditions discussed here. However, I am NOT an expert diagnostician of mental disorders. If ever you are in the slightest doubt always seek professional advice from those with the appropriate expertise.

I conclude with an insight arrived at by Bianca Acevedo and her team (2018) in their study comparing high sensitivity, autism, and other conditions: 'We suggest that adaptive SPS [or HSP] strategies involving empathy, awareness, calmness and physiological and cognitive self-control may serve a species by facilitating deep integration and memory for environmental and social information, which may ultimately foster survival, well-being, and cooperation.' HSPs' special gifts and essential place and purpose in this world are once again recognised and validated!

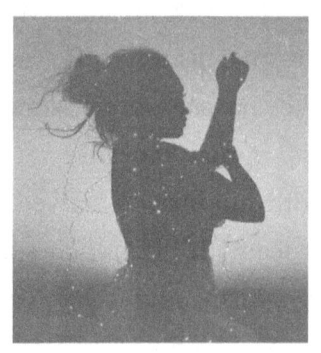

6

HSPs and Lifestyle

Balance

I believe the most important thing for all HSPs to address is getting the balance right between how much time they spend 'out there' in the world and how much time they spend in their own company in quiet retreat. As Elaine Aron (2001) puts it, you need to avoid being 'Out too much [and] in too much' (47). In other words, the question we have to answer for ourselves is how much and for how long do we open ourselves up to the elements (of our environment) and how much and for how long do we spend in refuge from them?

HSPs, like others, are easily enticed 'outside' and attracted to a world that constantly solicits their attention: the media, peer-group pressure, family expectations, social and cultural norms pull at us from all directions. Highly sensitive people are deeply affected by this. As I state in my book, *The Essential Flower Essence Book*

(2015), when describing those for whom Californian Poppy flower essence is useful:

> In this high-tech, speedy and hyper-stimulating world, it is very easy to be distracted and seduced. We can end up seeking outside ourselves for inspiration and false forms of higher consciousness, especially through escapism or addiction. Like a moth that is drawn to a light, we can easily become disorientated, exposed and vulnerable to predators and find ourselves burned or trapped by that which attracts us.

At work, HSPs experience the usual pressures to perform, to network and make a name for themselves, to develop 'their' brand etc. I wish I had a dollar for every time someone has said to me, 'Mark, you need to market yourself more aggressively!' My way would seem more low-key and laid back compared with many less sensitive people but I have learned that for the sake of my health and sanity it has to be that way! The truth is that my way of making my mark (pun intended) — and this is true for any HSP — can still be effective even if it isn't an extroverted approach. A prerequisite for career success for HSPs is that they need to know that what they are doing aligns with their values.

I have managed to make a good living, doing something that is meaningful and fulfilling for me while still attending to my needs as an HSP. I have done this by continuing to develop my skills and expertise as a naturopath throughout my career, ensuring that people are drawn to my practice by word of mouth and by writing and publishing books whose readership continues to increase.

For young HSPs there are social pressures from friends and peers to keep up with the crowd and not miss out on anything. But every day, HSPs need to have had enough downtime to be prepared for going out into the world, and after being 'out there' they need time to regroup. This fosters resilience.

Each HSP needs to find that balance between their social/outer life and personal/inner life without feeling pressured by others, especially those less comfortable in their own company. They, and even some professionals as mentioned in the previous chapter, may view this strong desire to spend time alone as something verging on a mental health issue. The fact is that if HSPs don't spend enough time in solitude they may well develop a mental issue! I cannot recall any HSP ever telling me that they felt lonely when they spend time alone — most have a rich inner life that for many includes a spiritual perspective that enhances their sense of connection with the wider world, so that they never really feel truly isolated. Occasionally, an HSP will realise that they've had too much 'alone-time' but this is rare because the social demands created by family, friends and work usually leave most HSPs craving more time to themselves.

Because of their sensitivity/reactivity to the dynamic 'atmospherics' of the world around them and the ease with which they can become overstimulated, HSPs need to be especially proactive in creating personal space. For many HSPs this involves:

- taking regular *time-outs* for rest and recovery and to reconnect with their inner strength and resources
- creating their *safe spaces* that have minimal stimulation and allow them to *calm*
- experiencing some solitude in which they can be 'nourished by their own thought processes and fantasies' (Ilse Sand, 2016)
- connecting with the *natural world* for energy replenishment and vitality.

Time *away from overstimulating environments* allows an HSP to move *into the depths of their perception*, where they are most comfortable and able to reconnect with inner strength and guidance.

Time Out

For HSPs, pausing to take time out is therapeutic on all levels. It soothes our souls! We need to remain aware of when we need to remove our overly sensitive selves from an overstimulating situation into one in which we can shed the dynamic, sometimes indelible, impression it has left on us. I recall describing to another highly sensitive person how, after visiting somewhere new or going to a party or dinner with friends, for the next 24 hours or so whenever I closed my eyes, in my mind's eye, I was back in that place again. She responded with a laugh: 'I thought I was the only one who did that! Whenever I've tried to describe it, people have looked at me as if I was a bit crazy. I feel so much better now I know there's someone else as mad as me!' (I was reassured too. The more people we meet who are 'mad' in the same way the less mad we feel!)

Regular time outs for highly sensitive people provide an opportunity for the stimulating sensations that have permeated their whole being to dissipate. Taking breaks enhances our natural resilience by allowing us to 'reboot' our system and then resume calm connections with others. As Ilse Sand says in her book *Tools for Helpful Souls*:

> Highly sensitive people can offer a connection and a form of presence that is of a very high quality. Many

of them are experts in providing a kind of empathic resonance that confirms the feelings of others and that can have a healing effect on them. They just can't do it for many hours at a time.

As someone once said to me by way of encouragement when I admitted to them that I desperately needed to take a break, 'That's fine with me, only rogues give more than they've got to give.'

There are a few HSPs who are able, through sheer willpower, to switch off and resist being overwhelmed even when surrounded by intense activity and noise. But they are the exception that proves the rule. And even if an HSP can use willpower in this way to stay 'out there' and perform for extended periods in very stimulating circumstances, invariably this comes at a cost — exhaustion and the need for extended time out for recovery. For other HSPs there are just some activities we need to 'psyche ourselves up' to do — shopping in a large and busy supermarket, for instance. But with careful planning and consideration such missions can be carried out successfully.

Here's how I do it. Firstly, plan a peaceful time-out for immediately after the mission is completed — get your priorities right! Secondly, commit to memory the list of products you need to buy and visualise in your mind exactly where these products are located in the aisles of the supermarket. Thirdly, when you arrive there, move swiftly through the aisles, changing lanes to avoid getting stuck behind shoppers who move at a snail's pace, seemingly on auto-pilot and mesmerised by their shopping experience. Next, once you have the required products in the bag make a b-line to the '12 items or less' lane at the checkout. Finally, if there are no annoying 'cheats' in the line in front of you with baskets containing more than twelve items, pay and make a quick escape. Feel the satisfaction of having successfully 'willed' yourself through the noise, the overstimulating lights and colours, the cold concrete floors, the electronic radiation, the nomadic browsers and aggressive, side-swiping shopping trolly drivers. Mission accomplished!

Calm and Safe Space

> *Living in harmony with others is always a challenge and it becomes more complicated when a person is highly sensitive by nature.*
>
> Maria Hill: www.sensitiveevolution.com

Often sensitive people develop a habit of attending to others' needs before their own, because they 'pick up' on discomfort around them and cannot feel comfortable themselves until others are settled. If they don't take time out to listen to their inner promptings, they find it difficult to get a sense of what their own needs are.

One of the keys to successfully negotiating the social world comes back to a tactic we have discussed — creating safe spaces to which we can retreat when necessary. I spoke earlier about my client Michael who learned as a child how to create personal spaces to which he could go when feeling overwhelmed, and how he carried this knowhow into his adult working life. This strategy allowed him to live in harmony, first with his family, and later with his work colleagues.

Another strategy that helps HSPs create a less stimulating and calmer space is to 'unclutter' their living and working environments. In an article called 'Why Highly Sensitive People Need Minimalism,' Melissa from the *Simple Lionheart Life* website (simplelionheartlife. com) states that one of the key benefits of minimalism for her is that it calms her as a Highly Sensitive Person:

> A lot of people feel stressed or unsettled in a cluttered environment. But Highly Sensitive People particularly feel the effects of chaos and clutter. Too much sensory information, including visual clutter, can easily make a Highly Sensitive Person feel overwhelmed and stressed.

And for those who begin to feel overwhelmed, anxious, and defeated by the idea of decluttering itself, the process doesn't need to be painful! Here are just two simple ways to begin:

1. Take the 12-12-12 Challenge. Locate 12 items in your house to throw away, 12 items to donate, and 12 items to be returned to their proper home — 36 things dealt with already! This could even be made into a quick competition between partner (and kids?) and you.
2. Give away one item each day. Colleen Madsen at '365 Less Things' gives away one item each day. Over the past several years, she has experienced quite a transformation simply by decluttering one day at a time.
http://www.oprah.com/spirit/why-you-must-have-solitude-and-time-for-yourself/all

Solitude

All of humanity's problems stem from man's inability to sit quietly in a room alone.
French scientist and philosopher Blaise Pascal, 1654.

HSPs are ahead of the game in regard to the their ability to 'sit quietly in a room alone'! As Ilse Sand (2016) says: 'Neither introverts nor sensitive people have a need for a lot of external stimuli ... [they] are nourished by their own thought processes and fantasies.'

I am not suggesting that highly sensitive people should lock themselves away in a room all day to daydream and fantasise! No, far from it, *highly sensitive people like everyone else need close connections with others*. However, most HSPs have learnt through necessity how important it is for their wellbeing to spend time alone so that, with a settled nervous system and a calm mind, they can regain perspective.

Many HSPs discover through experience that the secret to their resilience lies in making time to spend in quiet reflection, allowing them to reconnect with what many call the higher Self. Periods of quiet provide an opportunity to establish a point of inner stillness that can become a springboard for reorientation, refocus and redirection (see the chapter on Meditation). This passive/receptive state is extremely valuable in any decision-making process. In the midst of stress and overwhelm it is easy to make impulsive or muddled decisions that we may later regret. But anchored in a quiet interlude we can access the clarity of mind we need. 'Interlude' is a useful word in this context, with its connotations of a pause amid activity, part of a natural rhythmic order.

The Russian author and philosopher of the 19th century Fyodor Dostoevsky speaks highly of the beneficial effects of solitude, saying:

> [I find] solitude for the mind to be as essential as food is for the body. In solitude we can forge our character away from the constricting demands of others, and maintain our independence in the relationships we do cultivate, thus ensuring we do not, like many today, lose our identity in them.

Highly sensitive individuals need 'space' to consider their inner responses to the demands and subtle cues they experience from others around them. HSPs who do not work on aligning with the values most important to them through quiet, solitary reflection, may become too identified with the values and needs of others and be consumed by them. Thus they become less authentic, even though authenticity is a quality they rate so highly in themselves and others.

Far from being a sign that they are antisocial, solitude is constructive in helping HSPs to maintain high quality, authentic relationships. The quietened mind allows the highly sensitive person to replenish their energy and regain their poise so that when they re-engage with others, they can once more participate fully in their relationships.

The Natural World

As mentioned before, nature has an unusually beneficial soothing and calming effect on HSPs. Tapping into the plenitude of nature replenishes your vitality and provides soul food to strengthen the dynamic elements of your being. It improves resilience and enhances your natural immunity. I am not talking here about ingesting beneficial herbs or plants — we will discuss natural medicines later — but about connecting with the life force in nature through spending time in your garden, walking in your local park, visiting your refuge by the sea or just travelling out of the suburbs for some time spent in the countryside. Even looking briefly at pictures of the natural world can be refreshing and has, for example, been shown to increase the productivity of workers.

HSPs seem to benefit even more than others from spending time away from the human 'built-up' environment — the wider-than-human, natural world is particularly therapeutic for them. It is essential for me and many of my HSP clients to get out and commune in nature at least once a day. Five or ten minutes spent walking among the trees in a small park near my home always gives me a boost. As Dr Claire Henderson-Wilson from Victoria's Deakin University (2008) reminds us of how people are deeply connected to the natural environment emotionally, cognitively, aesthetically and even spiritually. This is especially true of HSPs. Being immersed in nature restores HSPs mentally when, as can easily happen, they suffer from sensory overload. According to Dr Henderson-Wilson, research suggests that a natural environment fosters recovery from mental fatigue caused by the overstimulation experienced by many urban residents — including all HSPs!

Quite simply, a green leafy outlook from your room or office is therapeutic. Research has shown that hospital patients whose beds have a view of green, growing things tend to heal faster and need less medication than those looking at a brick wall. Henderson-Wilson says people who spend 30 minutes or more in green spaces each week are less likely to experience high blood pressure or depression.

Here are some tips to help HSPs prevent or manage sensory overload:

1. Take your lunch break in a park or garden — away from your desk!
2. Go for walks or do your exercise outdoors.
3. If you are stuck inside, bring nature to you by surrounding yourself with indoor plants, and if at all possible, give yourself natural light exposure from a window with a 'green' view.
4. You can also bring nature to you by using natural medicines and therapies, as we will discuss later.

7

Health and Wellbeing for HSPs

Self-Care

Psychotherapist Ilse Sand (2016) believes that sensitive people rarely need to practice their empathic skills with others — they do it naturally. However, they do need to display more empathy towards themselves. They too often forget to focus on their own needs and feelings because they are so preoccupied with the needs and feelings of others around them. As an example from my own life, when my mother offered to throw a big 21st birthday party for me (a long time ago now!) I declined because I was too concerned about how people would get along with each other and whether they would enjoy themselves, etc. In hindsight I recognise a missed opportunity to have fun with my friends.

In order to make sense of their own intense emotional reactions, highly sensitive people need to create a personal space in which they can process them and be guided by them. At a deep level, emotions reveal information about our needs and values. According to the feelings-as-information theory (Schwartz, 2012), people utilise different feelings as sources of different types of information.

Emotions can be regarded as signals. As Frijda (1988, p. 354) states, 'emotions exist for the sake of signaling states of the world that have to be responded to, or that no longer need response and action.' In other words, emotions reveal important information about our interaction with the environment. For example, feelings of regret may inform us that we have not acted in line with how we believe we should or want to act. As such, emotions serve as a great source of information. The Positive Psychology Program B.V. (2019) states: 'By carefully listening to the information that an emotion signals to us, we can use this information to make choices and judgments that promote well-being' (141). In contrast, if an HSP becomes overwhelmed and loses their ability to use emotional information, their choices and judgments may be detrimental to their wellbeing.

Emotions have long been recognised as a means to communicate information about people's needs. Rosenberg (2003) defines the concept of needs as follows:

> [Needs] can be thought of as resources life

requires to sustain itself. For example, our physical wellbeing depends on our needs for air, water, rest, and food being fulfilled. Our psychological and spiritual wellbeing is enhanced when our needs for understanding, support, honesty and meaning are fulfilled ... all human beings have the same needs. Regardless of our gender, educational level, religious beliefs or nationality, we have the same needs. What differs from person to person is the strategy for fulfilling needs. (4)

Some examples of our needs include: choice, freedom, relatedness, competence, love, and closeness. In general, negative emotions indicate that a certain need is not being satisfied. Often the intensity with which emotion is felt by a highly sensitive person will mean that they don't respond immediately in proportion to it, to avoid conflict, for instance. The best approach is to pause, take time out and reflect. A commonly experienced state of mind for an HSP is tension, anxiety and stress from overstimulation, and this indicates a need for rest and relaxation. Positive emotions, on the other hand, signal that one's needs have been satisfied and that an activity (or non-activity in response to overstimulation) ought to be continued. Recognising your emotions as communicators of information about your needs will guide you in how to respond to them in practical ways. You can learn to be kind and properly care for yourself in this way.

An HSP's self-care list (to be ticked off!):

- Take more *responsibility for self* NOT just everything that happens around you.
- Make having frequent *times-to-self* a non-negotiable.
- Choose to do more of the *things you find pleasant* and less of the things you don't. (List your activities to make sure you have the right balance.)
- Engage in more activities you find *creative* — writing/reading, painting/sketching, craft, doing a crossword/puzzle, hobbies, etc. — activities in which you experience *flow*, a state of complete immersion.
- *Tune-up your body* with running, dancing, walking, swimming, bike-riding, bathing, palates, having a personal trainer, Naturopathy, Osteopathy, Chinese Medicine etc.
- *Nurture your body and soul* with Yoga, Tai chi, Relaxation exercise, Infra-red sauna and/or warmth of the sun, Meditation, etc.
- Spend time with *pets and animals* — cuddle, pat groom or walk them; or just BE with them.
- *Soothe your senses* with aromatherapy, music, making and eating healthy, nutritious and delicious

food, by having a massage (and/or exchanging one), by watching a relaxing movie or going to a classical music concert, for instance.
- *Immerse yourself in nature* by going for walks, hiking, spending time in the garden, surrounding yourself with plants, etc., or, if you can't always do this bring nature to you through healthy natural foods and eating behaviours, and natural medicines (refer later in chapter).
- Engage in *relationships* that feel meaningful, have depth and bring joy.

Drug Use

Many HSPs have used medications/drugs, prescribed or not, to numb their sensitivity. Human history is full of examples of highly sensitive, creative artists and performers who used drugs to calm, cope and manage their sensitivity. A number of my clients have used alcohol, for instance, to varying degrees as a way of managing the uncomfortable symptoms brought about by their high sensitivity when in social situations. As I learnt in my early adult years, at best it just puts off the inevitable realisation that you are more sensitive and need to live accordingly for your health's sake or, at worst, you suffer the damaging and cumulative effects of repeated minor trauma, though not aware of it at the time. The effect of a surgical anaesthetic is a good analogy — although you're not consciously aware of undergoing surgery, your body is still traumatised by it. I remember the excellent advice my surgeon gave me on my last day in hospital after undergoing open heart surgery to replace a faulty valve. I was 50 at the time and, buoyed by my speedy recovery I was a little overconfident as a result. The surgeon said to me: '

> Take it easy. Remember that your body still 'thinks' it's had a severe heart attack even though it was the surgery! You don't consciously remember any of it of course but your body is still, in effect, in recovery from what it experienced as serious trauma.

By my mid-20s I had chosen Natural Therapy approaches to enable me to live a more healthy, contented and productive life which would make room for my sensitivity and respect the depths of my feelings and perceptions. A good starting point was my GUT — giving much more consideration to what went into it, and how it was affected by my reactions to what was happening around me.

HSPs and Gut Health

My highly sensitive client Elizabeth consulted me one day about her digestive issues, saying:

> I am always trying to remember that I need to eat *in* comfort ... not *for* comfort! (laugh) ... If I am uncomfortable, or I'm in the wrong place or with people I don't wish to be with when I eat, I guarantee you I will get indigestion.

It is no surprise that highly sensitive people are prone to digestive problems if they eat while overstimulated — most people have this response! The problem is that HSPs are more *often* overstimulated, especially in company. When circumstances take any of us out of our comfort zone, the body's nervous system responds as it would to a perceived threat in the environment and prepares the body for fight or flight. There is increased blood flow to the muscles (to prepare for a powerful physical response) and a corresponding decreased blood flow to the intestinal organs, suppressing digestive function. Because HSPs are prone to being in this hypervigilant state, they need to give even more consideration to calming their nervous system before they eat. If they don't take measures to settle themselves down as much as possible, they will be susceptible to acute indigestion, and over the longer term, will develop chronic digestive issues.

Before Western Medicine established and promoted its understanding of the mechanisms that cause disease, doctors and healers in ancient traditions believed that many ailments were understood to originate from imbalances in the stomach/gut. Naturopathy, which was originally referred to as the 'Nature Cure,' has always emphasised the importance of gut health for general health and wellbeing. And indeed recent mainstream medical research into the gut microbiome to determine the type and balance of good and bad 'bugs' living in the gut has found a link between intestinal inflammation and chronic disease that supports this ancient understanding.

'Leaky Gut Syndrome' (LGS), a condition long recognised within Naturopathy, is gaining more recognition and acceptance in medical circles although it still has a way to go! Whether or not LGS ever finds a place in the medical dictionary (or finds its way there under another name!) the concept of compromised intestinal permeability and function is a useful one, and especially for HSPs.

Current research findings support the idea that inflammation resulting from modifications in intestinal bacteria plays a pivotal role in the development of acute digestive problems as well as chronic and systemic health issues. Increased intestinal permeability plays a role in certain gastrointestinal conditions such as irritable bowel syndrome (IBS), celiac disease, Crohn's disease, and, quite likely, many other auto-immune diseases.

In LGS the intestinal lining is compromised by increased permeability which allows partially digested food, toxins and gut flora to penetrate through to the tissues outside the gut. This can trigger inflammation and cause changes that lead to problems both within the digestive tract and outside in other tissues of the body.

When working properly, the lining of the gut is able to absorb nutrients from the food and drink you consume but does not absorb what is detrimental, toxic or not required. In other words, a healthy gut efficiently absorbs the good stuff and eliminates the bad stuff! Unhealthy food and drink, stress and emotional upset and also many medications can cause this natural process to falter. As food passes through our gastro-intestinal tract, sometimes the 'bad stuff' gets absorbed (or re-absorbed) through the intestinal lining and the 'good stuff' gets excreted before the gut absorbs the nutrients in it.

Everyone has some degree of leaky gut, as the gut needs to be permeable for it to perform its proper function. But severe cases of LGS are becoming more prevalent, along with other health issues that relate to a compromised gut lining. Modern life and a diet low in fibre and high in sugar and saturated fats may well be the main driver of increased gut inflammation in the general population. But some of us have a genetic predisposition to a digestive system that is more sensitive. HSPs, who are often keenly discerning and notice all the nuances in their environment, may be just as discerning about the food that enters their digestive system, responding acutely to nuances such as chemicals/additives, how food is processed, nutrient deficiencies etc. The gut portion of the gut-brain axis may well be as reactive as the brain part!

In my experience, sensitivity in an HSP commonly manifests systemically, expressing itself on physical levels in the form of environmental allergies, gut 'sensitivities' and intolerances, a 'nervous gut' etc. Because highly sensitive people are more prone to becoming overstimulated, emotionally upset and mentally overwhelmed it is not surprising that the gut is affected, especially if they eat at these times. If you are overwhelmed and not able to properly 'digest' what is going on *around* you, how can you expect to properly digest what is going *into* you? It is no wonder then that life can easily give you indigestion!

Our gut and brain do communicate, and some people, especially HSPs, hear what their gut has to 'say' loud and clear! This gut-brain axis consists of bi-directional communication between the central nervous system and the enteric nervous system which directly controls gastrointestinal function. This axis links the emotional and cognitive centers of the brain with the functions of our gut. I have spoken often in this book about how most HSPs (including myself) have come to rely heavily on understanding gut responses to our immediate environment — for safety, guidance and generally navigating the world.

Highly sensitive people's gut health is of primary importance because we use our gut responses as guidance in this way. When gut health is compromised, or when we become overstimulated to the point of being overwhelmed, we HSPs can temporarily lose our ability to properly read our innate emotional compass, the thing that helps us navigate safely and calmly through life.

As mentioned, a properly balanced gut microbiota (gut flora balance) is extremely important for optimum function of gut-brain communication and general health and wellbeing. There is a strong link between the gastrointestinal microbiota and brain structure and function. Here are some ways to improve and/or maintain balanced and healthy gut flora (microbiota):

- Remove foods that can be inflammatory and/or that promote changes in gut flora — the most

common culprits are sugar/alcohol, gluten, dairy, food additives/chemicals and many processed foods. Avoid the foods to which you are allergic, sensitive or to which you show intolerance.
- Be aware that many prescribed medications have a negative impact on our bowel flora. Antibiotics, for instance, wipe out the 'nasty' flora but also eliminate much of the beneficial/healthy flora. (Consult your professional health practitioner for advice on appropriate probiotics.)
- Incorporate some healthy fermented foods into your diet, such as sauerkraut, kefir, kombucha, miso, tempeh, yoghurt (if OK with dairy).
- Eat unprocessed and seasonal foods as much as possible.
- As important as any of the above is to always try to create the most comfortable and relaxed environment for yourself when you eat. Avoid eating when you are emotionally upset — it can spoil the benefits of a perfectly healthy meal! A calm and mindful state will always promote the best digestive outcome for you.

Finally, I know how grateful HSP clients have been when I have been able to help them alleviate their gut and digestive problems through my Naturopathic work with them. I strongly advise anyone to seek professional guidance in this area. After all, our gut is part of our brain and is therefore so important for clarity of awareness in HSPs. Keep it healthy and functioning at its optimum!

Western Medical Approaches

A clinical setting can be an uninviting and cold environment that makes HSPs feel uncomfortable. White coat hypertension (WHT), more commonly known as white coat syndrome, is something I experience when I visit my General Practitioner, despite her calm, empathic and in no way threatening demeanour. This response is also experienced by many other, less sensitive people. Frequently the 'atmosphere' of a medical practice or hospital clinic is not an ideal space for an HSP to calmly and clearly articulate their health concerns — rising anxiety levels can quickly lead to overwhelm.

In many medical practices, large patient numbers create time constraints which means there is a greater sense of urgency and exclusive focus on detecting potentially life-threatening and serious health signs and symptoms. It is no wonder that HSPs often tell me they don't feel 'heard' or understood in medical environments. Most of the time it is no reflection on the medical doctor's competence or willingness to help — it is the mismatch of this clinical environment with sensitivity that is the problem. HSPs are more likely to feel heard and understood when their intuition and self-awareness can be used to clearly articulate their concerns. This is made easier when appreciated by a doctor who can take advantage of this valuable information.

Many HSPs experience subjective symptoms that are not a 'good fit' with Western Medical Diagnoses. Idiosyncratic signs and symptoms may not be easily assigned to a specific medical condition or disorder, may be misunderstood and wrongly assigned, or worse, just dismissed as unimportant and of no value.

HSPs also often experience strong responses to clinical doses of medications, including experiencing more numerous and more intense physiological side-effects. Anecdotally many of my clients have shared with me that they respond better to 'subclinical' doses of medications. Less is better (and this can also apply to natural remedies, so see below).

Make your practitioner aware of your sensitivity!

I am not for one moment implying that you should ever hesitate to consult your doctor if you have any concerns about your health. Their life-saving expertise and skills are not in question here. I have written the above to provide important considerations for HSPs to take into account when choosing their doctors.

Traditional and Complementary Medical Approaches
The philosophies underpinning traditional therapies such as TCM (Traditional Chinese Medicine), Naturopathy, Ayurvedic Medicine, Herbal Medicine etc. are based on the understanding that the body possesses an inherent ability to heal itself. Methods used by these natural therapy approaches to overcoming illness are therefore those that restore and promote the body's own normal and OPTIMUM function. Advice, guidance and natural medicines are tailored to the individual's needs based on a holistic view of the person. For example, on my website, hsphealth.com.au, I describe how the natural medicines used in my practice are:

1. Safe and without side-effects — *Non-Toxic*
2. Assist and enable the body to heal itself — *Non-Dependence Forming*
3. Encourage the body to function at its optimum (not just be symptom free) — *Improve Health and Wellbeing*

I have also come to understand that many HSPs seek out Natural Therapies because:

- As mentioned above, HSPs often experience strong responses to clinical doses of medications, including more numerous, and more intense, physiological side-effects. As a consequence, they are very receptive to complementary medical approaches to health management which are generally less invasive and more subtle in their action (for example Flower Essences, Herbal Medicines, etc.) But even with natural medicines HSPs often respond better to 'subclinical' doses — using a smaller dose works best for them. For instance, I find that lower doses of a Vitamin B Complex work best for calming my nervous system, whereas the more commonly recommended larger doses tend to 'hype' me up. That is an HSP for you!
- Symptoms experienced by HSPs are frequently not a 'good fit' with Western medical diagnoses, often being unique and highly subjective. These idiosyncratic signs and symptoms can be difficult to assign to a specific condition or disorder within the medical model.
- HSPs frequently feel that they have not been 'heard' or understood in a clinical medical context. Time constraints understandably force medical practitioners to focus, in the short time they have,

on eliminating the possibility of a life-threatening condition. This often results in an approach that does not provide the ideal time and space for an HSP to calmly and clearly articulate their health concerns.
- There is also little time (or motivation) for a medical practitioner to listen to or take advantage of the self-awareness-based information that could be provided by an HSP. If heard at all, the HSP may be written off as merely anxious or neurotic. By contrast, the subjective symptoms that differentiate an individual's experience from that of others (even with the same diagnosed medical condition) are of prime importance to most alternative medical practitioners when making their assessment. HSPs commonly do feel heard in this context, when their self-knowledge is appreciated. They feel validated.

Natural Medicine(s) for HSPs

There are many natural medicines and natural approaches that can help and support the health and wellbeing of a highly sensitive person. To cover them in detail is for another book! However, there is one composite natural remedy that I feel all highly sensitive persons can benefit from knowing about. It is a remedy that has played a huge role in my life in helping me to manage my high sensitivity. It has also been a standout and stand-alone remedy in my practice as a Naturopath and Counsellor. I have prescribed it to literally thousands of clients, and for many it has become their 'go to' tool as a highly sensitive person. The natural remedy is produced by Flower Essence Services (FES) in Nevada, USA and it is called YES (Yarrow Environmental Solution) flower essence formula.

YES is a unique and potent blend of flower essences and plant tinctures in a sea-salt water base to help strengthen and protect against *toxic environmental influences*. For me, and for many of my clients, it acts like a dynamic, personal bodyguard! The YES formula was originally developed by the Flower Essence Society in response to Russian health practitioner requests after the Chernobyl nuclear disaster in 1986. Kaminski and Katz (1994) inform us that YES 'directly counteracts the destructive effects of radiation on the human energy field.' All the herbs used in the formula have a reputation for enhancing *natural immune response*. When combined, their *synergistic effect* amplifies their ability to strengthen *natural immunity on all levels*.

> The purpose of YES formula is to strengthen and protect against toxic environmental influences, geopathic stress and other hazards of modern

life. These include the effects of radiation from x-rays, televisions, computer monitors, cell phones, electromagnetic fields, radiation treatments and cosmic radiation to which we are exposed during high-altitude flights. Many practitioners use it as a baseline remedy and ongoing stabiliser when addressing fundamental health issues endemic to the modern world. (Wells 2016, *The Essential Flower Essence Book*)

The YES formula acts as a strong energetic shield to help protect against 'environmental challenges to wellbeing and vitality; strengthening and protecting' (Patricia Kaminski, FES co-director).

From an emotional sensitivity perspective, a star component of the YES formula is the Pink Yarrow flower essence. It is a remedy that I frequently prescribe on its own (or with YES) for self and other clients when the integrity of one's 'emotional boundaries' need to be secured. All plants of the Yarrow family *protect against negativity* in the immediate environment. Pink Yarrow enhances this 'protective' quality in relation to those with whom there is an *emotional attachment* or vested interest — family, loved ones, friends and clients. It acts like an energetic *emotional buffer* between us and others — *emotional boundaries* become better defined. In other words, it helps us to recognise who is feeling what — being able to discern between *my stuff* (what *I'm* feeling) and *your stuff* (what *you're* feeling) in relationships. Pink Yarrow protects against taking on other people's *negative emotions*, something that HSPs constantly grapple with. In summary:

> Pink Yarrow's negative signs:
> Overly sympathetic — 'psychic sponge'
> Lacking emotional boundaries (FES)
>
> Pink Yarrow's benefits:
> 'Self-contained consciousness' (FES) while maintaining empathy
> Emotional clarity

8
....

Work, Career and Vocation

Which jobs suit a highly sensitive person?

It can take a long time for highly sensitive people to feel comfortable in the workplace, and many change jobs and try different things until they find their niche. There are many niches that are not the best fit, such as jobs in which we can never be alone or where the work environment is too noisy. My client Jasmine quite liked aspects of her original job but those aspects she didn't like became overwhelming in the end. Her sensitivity to her work environment meant that she was constantly overstimulated, leaving her with no energy for her life outside work.

> There are some parts of my previous job that I really miss. A couple of good friends that I don't see too often now. Also, I was pretty much given free rein to do my own thing — graphic designing, making

short videos, helping with website design etc. for us and our clients. But, unfortunately, we worked in an open office situation. The background noise and activity were big distractions for me — loud music at times, people talking loudly and moving around all the time, bright lights, no decent outside views. I would come home exhausted. My health eventually suffered. The new job I have now allows me to work from home a lot — a generally quiet space for me to be creative! I seem to have got the balance right for now. I won't think too far ahead though — or maybe I should! — because my partner and I are thinking of starting a family. At least I've worked out a few things before we start!

More than two out of three Australians value happiness over money, and more than half believe that meaningful work is more important than salary — although money is often a close second! I have no doubt that the percentage of HSPs who value meaningful work over salary would be even greater.

Elaine Aron (1996) suggests that if you are to thrive at work you need to 'Follow your bliss and let your light shine through.' She says that much of HSPs' difficulty at work results from 'not appreciating [their] role, style and potential contribution' on the one hand, and on the other, a need to 'understand and appreciate ... [their] vocation's place in [their] rich, inner world — its deeper MEANING for [them]' (116).

HSPs need meaningful work where their contribution is valued. I'm not suggesting that recognising your vocation or 'calling' (in its widest sense) is easy. But for most HSPs this is at least an essential aspiration. When seeking clarity about suitable work people so often seek outside guidance and often get it from well-meaning but perhaps less sensitive people who are often the first to come forward with advice. This advice may be very useful and practical for the majority but not so for HSPs.

Traditional career counselling involves matching someone's abilities and interests with job characteristics. This may be of little use to HSPs. For them, 'identifying their most deeply held values, and planning life goals which actualise those values may be the treatment of choice. Career development then becomes the search for meaning rather than the search for a job; (Jaeger, 2004, 110). Back in the 1970s and 1980s, during the dawn of the so-called New Age, 'personal growth' workshops and courses were common. The best thing I got from participating in one was discovering my vocation through identifying my values as described above. Once I had done this, I planned life goals that would enable me to actualise those values. (I had chopped and changed jobs on a regular basis up until that moment!) Then as now, living my values gives me my sense of purpose and meaning, having found that the best answers lay at the heart of my being. As Carl Jung put it, 'Who looks outside, dreams; who looks inside, wakes.'

Dr Barrie Jaeger puts it this way: 'Grow yourself and your real work will grow towards you. This is what the sensitive person needs to do' (2004, 11). Dr Jaeger is an expert in vocational guidance, especially for HSPs, and stresses the importance of understanding yourself and your needs as a highly sensitive person. This self-acceptance allows you to 'look at the bigger picture of how you experience work as a Sensitive Person' (12). This way you will avoid the jobs that don't work for you and, ultimately, find your true calling and discover work that brings joy, creativity and a high level of satisfaction.

In the meantime, take pride in what Dr Elaine Aron (2001) states about HSPs, pointing out that they are:

> highly conscientious, loyal, vigilant about quality, good with details, intuitive visionaries, often gifted, thoughtful of the needs of clients or customers, and good influences on the social climate of the workplace ... [making] ideal employees. Every organisation needs some. (236)

The environment in which an HSP works is as important as the type of work they engage in. In the next chapter we describe the best work environments.

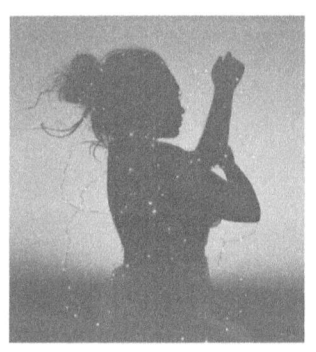

9

Ideal Environments for HSPs

Generally, a person with high sensitivity will prefer an environment that does not overstimulate them. As mentioned earlier, HSPs usually start from a point of higher arousal to begin with — they may hover around the moderate to high range even when very little is happening around them. So it doesn't take much extra stimulation for HSPs to reach a point of over-arousal, a state of sensory overwhelm that affects their ability to function at their best. Over-arousal can be prevented through self-management — using time-outs, meditation, etc. — and management of their immediate environment.

In this chapter, we will go into more detail about how an HSP can better manage their immediate environment so they can establish their ideal home and work-space. I will use Dr Annemarie Lombard's (2014) term 'environmental goodness of fit' — 'how people and the environment relate to one another to produce a positive or negative outcome ... when there is an optimum fit between the individuals and their environment based on their sensory needs, they thrive, enjoy life and are productive' (109).

HSPs at Home

Here is a checklist of the WORST environmental factors for HSPs at home, as described by thousands of my highly sensitive clients over the years. They won't all apply to everybody, but most HSPs will recognise them:

- Loud noise, bright lighting, strong odours, excessive use of intense and stimulating colour in decor
- Cluttered space
- Change/unpredictability in immediate surroundings — constant re-arrangement of furniture/living spaces and creation of mess
- Inability to regulate temperature, 'stuffy'/thick atmosphere
- Excessive radiation from televisions, computer monitors and equipment (including routers — they are part of life now but at least consider turning them off at bedtime and/or don't sleep within their vicinity), cell phones, household appliances etc.
- No designated quiet time/personal space area and/

or a bedroom in noisiest area of house — next to living/entertainment room, for instance
- Entertaining large groups of people
- Apartment-living with shared walls lacking sound barriers
- Lack of natural light, lack of natural views / harsh urban-only views
- No secluded garden space
- Built-up, busy, noisy part of city/town
- Geopathic stress from surroundings — signal towers, electric power lines, other electromagnetic fields
- Need to travel excessive distances to work

Here on the other hand is a checklist for BEST environmental fit at home:

- Quiet, calming decor
- Minimalist approach — uncluttered, spacious (but contained), clean lines, a restrained palette and simplicity
- Good temperature regulation, ventilated
- Minimum TV, computer equipment etc., all confined to one area in home
- Designated quiet and personal space
- Bedroom in quietest area of home

- Small and intimate groups of people if entertaining
- Good sound barriers between inside and outside house, e.g. double glazed windows, shared walls soundproofed
- Lots of natural light and views of nature
- Secluded garden space
- Quiet part of city/town
- Low geopathic stress from signal towers, electric power lines, other electromagnetic fields
- Close to work — minimal travelling

HSPs at Work

Most factors that provide the best environmental fit at home for HSPs as described above can also be applied to the workplace. Some more specific points related to work and work relationships are made below.

Checklist for BEST environmental fit at work:

- Aim for the lowest possible level of stimulation — QUIET AND CALM surroundings work best for HSPs
- Sit where you feel comfortable — a bit to the side, not centrally and away from the activity hub. Avoid sitting under an air conditioning vent!

- Keep your space clean, neat and organised — a 'minimalist' approach generally works best.
- Rely mostly on natural lighting — your desk by a window with a view of nature, for instance.
- Find a space with muted or pastel colours.
- Reduce glare from your computer screen and use a blank screen saver.
- Turn down the ringtone volume on your phone and reduce/remove other auditory distractions (discreet use of ear plugs may be useful when noise levels rise).
- Structure quiet breaks/downtime into your workday — 'green' time outside is best and essential!
- As mentioned, always aspire to work as close to home as possible (or work from home). I find my short walk to and from work one of the simple pleasures in life!

Make sure your employer is aware of the following:

- You don't work as well when being observed for the purpose of evaluation and would prefer other means of evaluating your performance (see Aron, 2001).
- Aggressive self-promotion takes you way out of your comfort zone. You would just like to be

recognised and respected for the quality of your work and the honest and diligent way you go about it.
- You thrive on being provided with clear expectations, structure and predictability.

10

HSPs in Relationships

The major purpose of this book is to help HSPs embrace their gift of high sensitivity, appreciate their essential place and the contribution they make in the world, and generally feel good about themselves. If we don't like and respect ourselves how can we expect others to? On the other hand, if we *do* like and respect ourselves, it is much easier for others to do the same. Loving and fulfilling relationships are the result.

We know that HSPs have to find the right balance between being 'out there' in the world and spending time alone 'in their world.' The same applies in personal relationships. HSPs must get the balance right between how much time they spend engaging fully with their partner/loved one/friend and how much time they spend alone or doing their own thing. This invariably requires a 'less sensitive' partner to gain a deeper understanding of what it means to be highly sensitive.

Many less sensitive people may initially think that their HSP friend's need for time alone indicates a lack of interest or commitment to the relationship or, at worst, signifies rejection. They may come to a similar conclusion when an HSP suddenly needs to leave a social event early, or just doesn't wish to socialise at all on some occasions. One could easily take offence if they don't understand that their highly sensitive friend is just taking a very necessary time out in order to bounce back resiliently and be fully attentive and the best company tomorrow or the next time they meet.

Less sensitive friends and family may also need to learn that HSPs' response to stress or trauma, for instance, may often be to spend *more* time alone, not less. I had open heart surgery at the age of 50 to correct a faulty aortic heart valve, first discovered in my teens. The weeks immediately after open heart surgery are difficult for anyone (HSP or not). In order to survive and best recover during that time, my prime focus had to be to create and maintain adequate personal SPACE! Being in our home as a single parent to two teenagers, with no partner to 'shield' me from well-meaning well-wishers, I had to be brutally honest on some occasions with loved ones and friends about my desperate need to grab what time alone I could.

Being an HSP, in those initial weeks after surgery I

found it doubly tiring to be with people — one because of my sensitivity, and two, because of my vulnerable condition. Inevitably there were friends who took it personally when I seemed to reject them. But it was about survival for me, so I had no choice. It was interesting in hindsight when I recognised that most of those who were understanding and *didn't* feel aggrieved were the more sensitive (and more introverted) among my friends — the very ones who normally do feel things very deeply! This must also say something about where empathy stems from.

Another point I will make here is that as an HSP, I was actually asking for *less* contact/assistance, not more, in order to get through a difficult period in my life. This directly contradicts the misguided view some people have, that HSPs are 'high maintenance' in the workplace or at home. High sensitivity does not equate with being excessively needy!

If an HSP is in a relationship with a less sensitive and very needy person, this is potentially problematic. If someone is very demanding and needs to be with their highly sensitive partner at all times, the HSP will either become emotionally exhausted or will try desperately to find some personal space, or both. The less sensitive person will need to accept this and allow the HSP some personal space, even just by being in different rooms of the house at times! Often that is all the highly sensitive person needs — HSPs are very resilient if given half a chance.

What an HSP Brings to Relationships

Some of the same points (plus a few others) used in Chapter 2 to describe common characteristics of a highly sensitive person are used in the following to illustrate some of the positive qualities that a HSP brings to any relationship.

- HSPs are *concerned about the world* and everyone and everything in it. Highly sensitive people care for themselves and all human and non-human creatures, feeling a deep connection to everything around them. This connection means they care about and are very aware of any impact they have on their surroundings and the people in it. Anyone in relationship with an HSP will always sense that care and concern.

- HSPs are *inclined to 'feel' their way* through life. They know what it is like to feel deeply, especially when feelings are uncomfortable and painful. They *are able to remember how it feels*, so they are careful with the feelings of others. Their natural empathy means they are sensitive to and in tune with the way others are feeling. It is a great skill and reflects their good emotional and social IQ. Anyone in relationship with an HSP will be a beneficiary.

- HSPs bring their *passion, search for meaning and sense of spirituality* to a relationship. By *spirituality* here I mean a rich inner world, one that often prompts them to express a unique and imaginative viewpoint. They have a unique vision, understanding and approach to any given situation that makes HSPs interesting and entertaining to be with. But when a highly sensitive person uses this unique perspective to express or produce something with deep *meaning* and exhibit it with *passion,* something great can be created for all those around.

- HSPs are *good at noticing nuances* and are *cautious and consider their options*. This allows them to actively observe and utilise their intuitive ability which has taught them to understand people in an entirely different way. Thinking (and sometimes standing) 'outside the square,' a highly sensitive person can often conceive novel solutions to deal with problems and conflicts. They are skilled at avoiding making comments, especially during heated discussions, that may inflame a situation. This is one of their survival skills because most HSPs find conflict very uncomfortable.

- HSPs are authentic, and just as they are not interested in engaging for any length of time in shallow, superficial conversation, they are also not too interested in talking about themselves or others in a shallow or superficial way. It must surely have been two HSPs who came up with the phrase 'we need to have a deep and meaningful'! For sensitive people it seems natural to share deeper, more authentic insights about themselves and operating through a persona manufactured for public consumption will exhaust them — and they *need to conserve energy.* Also, through much self-reflection, they often come to accept who they are and don't feel the need to present fake personalities. Sincerity is a strong character trait and something that HSPs respect but also 'crave' from others. For this reason, they will go out of their way to create the opportunity and space for other people to share their deeper nature. HSPs know too well how important it is for one's wellbeing to be able to 'open up' occasionally in a safe space!
- HSPs are generally unselfish. I have found that one of the reasons many highly sensitive people desire to spend time on their own is because, when in company, their instinctive response is outwards, towards the other. Hence many cannot ever

completely rest until they spend time alone. Highly sensitive people are born with a predisposition to over-respond to sensations from the environment (Lombard, 2014). Selfishness, or any type of self-centredness in relation to others goes against the grain for a sensitive person — their prime focus is on the other and it causes them distress to ignore others' needs in favour of their own. Most sensitive people have a great sense of responsibility and are *highly responsive* to people and the world around them.

HSPs in Relationships

I highly recommend you read Annemarie Lombard's book (2014), "Sensory Intelligence — why it matters more than IQ or EQ", especially the Chapter 4 on "Sensory intelligent relationships" (pg. 89).

For a highly sensitive person to be happy, content and grow in their relationships they need to:

- Make sure they get enough 'alone-time.'
- Discuss their need for balance between social activity and solitude with partner.
- Create their personal space where they can be alone — this may even include separate beds or bedrooms.
- Have quiet space away from activity, TV, radio etc.

- Deal with one issue at a time.
- Remain aware of their tendency to take everything personally — be alert to any of their over-reaction and give themselves time to settle.
- Learn how to ask for what they need.
- Have a no-yelling rule — heated conflict 'burns' any HSPs in the vicinity!
- Avoid overly people-pleasing and appeasing, and especially don't try to fix your partner.
- Discuss the need to respect bathroom time.
- Have some fun!

HSP in relationship with another HSP

Advantages:
- Your needs are similar and you understand each other
- You 'keep the peace' and minimise the sensory input within your home and your lives
- You make your home a secure, harmonious space
- Quiet time together is enjoyable and satisfying in itself

Challenges:
- Both of you can easily become too structured, rigid and controlling, losing any spontaneity

- If you become set in your ways, compromise becomes an issue — you lose the ability to adapt to change
- At least one of you may need to become the catalyst to venture out of your comfort zone and explore new activities and social interactions to guard against withdrawing too much from society. You still need to strike the right balance between time 'out there' in the world and time spent by yourselves.

HSP in relationship with non-HSP

Advantages:
- The less sensitive partner will challenge the highly sensitive partner to be more social, venture out and explore in the world, and not get too set in their ways.
- The highly sensitive partner will be a stabilising influence on the less sensitive partner, helping them to establish the right balance between calm, peaceful time out with less sensory input, and other highly stimulating activities.

Challenges:

- The sensory needs of each partner are completely different: 'Their respective pursuit and avoidance of sensation can create a lot of friction, irritation and conflict' (Lombard, 2014). ** For example, the less sensitive partner wants to try a new restaurant (getting sick of the same old same old!), while the HSP wants to stay with their tried and proven restaurant where the food and ambience are just right, and best of all there will be no surprises!
- The less sensitive partner can get 'high' on being busy, loud, talkative and 'abuzz.' Just being in their presence can create sensory overload and overwhelm the HSP.
- The less sensitive partner may be reluctant to try to understand high sensitivity, or worse may believe it is a weakness that should be changed. It is easier for the highly sensitive person to understand the needs of a less sensitive person, as they are much more overtly expressed.

**Identify and prioritise the things you do have in common — common needs, things you both enjoy doing, etc.

11

Meditation for HSPs

Thomas Moore, author of *Care of the Soul* (1992), sums up a common problem when he says:

> We seem to have a complex about 'busyness' in our culture. Most of us do have time that we could devote to simple relaxation, but we convince ourselves that we don't.

And, if we do recognise that we have some time up our sleeve to relax, we feel guilty about spending time idly, thinking we should be doing something. Dr Ainslea Meares describes how a highly sensitive person, who can become over-stimulated easily, would benefit from making time for relaxation:

> The most important thing that we can do in helping our brain integrate the excess of impulses which it

is receiving is to let our mind run quietly for a while. (*Life Without Stress*, 1987)

When an HSP's mind is allowed to 'run quietly,' an ability innate in all of us, it will not only reduce stimulus overload in the brain, but also help the brain to work more efficiently. Ainslie Meares, a psychiatrist and hypnotherapist who practised in Melbourne from the 1930s till the 1980s, believed that if we allow ourselves to reconnect with this ability, we can experience what he called 'atavistic regression' — a biologically primitive mental state in which the mind does not register discomfort or emotion of any kind.

This practice of achieving atavistic regression is now referred to as Stillness Meditation Therapy (SMT) through the work of Pauline McKinnon, author of a number of books on the subject. She gave this practice of deep mental relaxation its name and has remained dedicated to teaching it through individual consultations, group sessions and SMT teacher training courses in which I have participated. She was originally a patient of Dr Meares and has remained true to his way of experiencing meditation. Inner quiet, which is needed for meditation, is eventually established through persistence and by a non-judgmental acceptance of thoughts and feelings, allowing them to pass further and further into the background. When such inner calm is achieved even fleetingly, a profound *stillness* can reveal itself, and in this state of rest, the mind's own powers of healing can be activated. If we regularly experience this state of mind through the practice of meditation, it provides a quiet and still mental platform from which we can function, free of overwhelm and stress, in our everyday life.

More than most, HSPs recognise our human need for refuge or time out from our increasingly complex and stimulating lifestyle. The problem is that this same lifestyle provides few quiet places of retreat where we can feel safe and secure, and responsibilities to family, friends and society can keep us constantly on the go. Meanwhile, we are assaulted by noise and other sensory stimulation from the outside world. When we do get away from it all and by chance find some peaceful oasis in our day, the *internal* racket our minds create can be even more problematic via overwhelming, erratic and negative thought processes. Our struggle for inner silence and stillness of mind is often mirrored by a parallel struggle to tune out *external* noise and stimuli. However, if we practise meditation on a regular basis the struggle becomes less and a calmness of mind increasingly permeates our day.

At the age of 20, many years before I came across the term HSP, I was fortunate enough to be given a copy of

Ainslie Meares's book (1970), *Relief Without Drugs*. At that stage, I had already suffered from migraines since childhood. I was aware that my high level of nervous tension through an inability to fully relax physically and mentally was an important factor in the migraines' persistent recurrence. Dr Meares's book, which was first published way back in 1967, made great sense to me. I soon started regularly practising the stillness meditation (SMT) he described.

Without wanting to sound too dramatic, I do wonder whether I would be alive today if I had not started practising this form of relaxation/meditation all those years ago. As mentioned in earlier chapters, I have a significant family history of heart disease and until my mid-twenties had engaged in binge drinking in an attempt to numb my high sensitivity. Meditation not only improved my quality of life but also extended it! One of the mantras I repeat over and over to my clients is: 'If you concentrate on achieving a good quality of life, you will achieve a good quantity of life!'

As mentioned, my first experience of meditation in my early twenties was the type promoted by Dr Ainslie Meares. During my mid to late twenties, I tried other meditation approaches, some from the Buddhist tradition and also Transcendental Meditation (TM). They certainly weren't wasted experiences and kept me inspired to maintain a regular meditation practice. From my early 30s though, I returned to Stillness Meditation and have maintained this practice ever since. Some years later, Mindfulness meditation became accepted by the mainstream health community. I studied and facilitated Mindfulness groups as a component of my Masters in Social Science (Human Relations/Counselling). Through all that time I also continued my Stillness Meditation practice. I always found, and research supports my experience, that mindfulness is a natural biproduct of meditation.

Stillness Meditation (SMT) has a 'goodness of fit' with HSPs

I am fully aware of the benefits brought to millions around the world by various styles of meditation and mindfulness, but from my own experience as a regular meditator, teacher of meditation, and observer of clients' responses, I strongly recommend Stillness Meditation Therapy for HSPs for the following reason(s). Most HSPs are already in a naturally mindful state in the sense that they are acutely aware of what's going on around and within them whether they like it or not! As my highly sensitive client Cassandra put it in her initial consultation with me:

I never miss the sounds of the world waking in the morning because they have usually woken me up! I automatically notice the world around me, all the sounds, colours and smells. I only wish I could have a break from them sometimes! I'm always aware of feelings, especially the feelings of others which I do my best not to take on. I always notice the tone of someone's voice, their subtle mannerisms, and with some, the draining effect they have on me. And I know it sounds bad but sometimes I quite literally feel a pain in my bum when I can't get away from some people!

Natural medicine and regular practice of Stillness Meditation has worked beautifully for Cassandra over time!

HSPs are constantly drawn into a present moment awareness because of their natural vigilance and attention to detail. When in a balanced state they appreciate, absorb and reflect on sensations and subtle environmental cues that would normally go unnoticed by those less sensitive. When out of balance, however, this intensity of experience, as discussed in previous chapters, can lead to becoming overwhelmed and stressed. At such times, mindfulness practices can create further stimulation by increasing their already acute awareness of what's around them, contributing to further sensory overload. Stillness Meditation Therapy works extremely well for many highly sensitive people because it tends to bypass external awareness focus and move directly and effortlessly inward towards calm and the experience of stillness.

SMT as taught by Ainslie Meares is characterised by its ABSENCE OF TECHNIQUE — there are no mantras, no music, no chanting, no visualisations, no breathwork and no rituals. SMT transcends these 'techniques' through an effortless experience where people return to a natural state of being with a mind at rest, undisturbed by discomfort and thoughts. When SMT is understood and practised regularly, outcomes include reduced anxiety and stress, preventing entirely or avoiding relapses into other conditions such as depression. Stillness Meditation is about *not* doing or focusing on anything. All that's required to gain the full benefits of SMT is regular practice. As Pauline McKinnon puts it, 'There is a discipline to it, but not a technique.'

SMT and other types of meditation truly can be life-changing, and their particular usefulness for HSPs is that regular practice has a 'flow on' effect into the rest of their day. The regular experience of stillness and inner calm gained from practice means that it becomes a familiar state of being that is more and more readily accessible just by thinking about it at other times. This then enables the highly sensitive person to adapt and cope better with whatever circumstances may arise.

Meditation for highly sensitive children and adolescents

Infants and very young children have a natural ability to relax and let go of tension. It is usually only as they get older and begin school that they begin losing touch with this ability. In teaching highly sensitive children meditation we can keep them connected with their inner calm, stillness and strength, helping them to keep it at hand as they get older (when it is needed most!)

For adolescents, meditation can be introduced as a positive life skill to assist in lowering anxiety/stress and performing at their best. We have already discussed how highly sensitive people demonstrate vantage sensitivity and so respond even better than other less sensitive people to any positive intervention. The practice of meditation, skilfully introduced into a class situation for instance, empowers kids — their confidence develops, resilience builds, relationships improve, studies flourish. Independent thought is cultivated that protects against being too influenced by peers and the media, or too reliant on alcohol, drugs etc. It helps bring an inner calm to a time of life when there is pressure to be productive and to achieve.

Finally, HSPs experience intense emotions constantly and meditation is about practising acceptance of these emotions so that the important messages they convey can be understood. If we try to push away or deny our strong feelings they will only intensify and the overwhelm felt means the message is lost. All our feelings are valid and their acceptance is crucial to self-validation.

Psychologist Rick Hanson's description (from his website: www.rickhanson.net) of what he calls a *mindful* person — a consequence of meditation — also describes the perception of the world experienced by HSPs when they are at ease and relaxed:

> You perceive more fully, seeing the big picture, putting things in perspective. You free up energy that was spent pushing down your real feelings. You tune into your body, your heart. You're less fixed or attached in your views. You recognize the good things in you and around you that you'd tuned out. You feel more supported, more protected. You take things less personally. You feel at home in yourself.
>
> **Dr Rick Hanson**

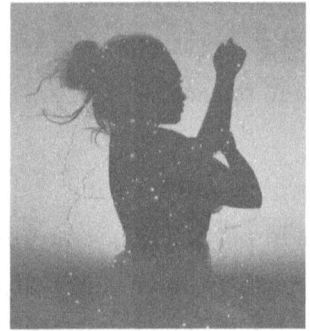

12

HSPs and Spirituality

Human Perceptions are not bounded by organs of Perception: a human-being perceives more than sense can discover. (Neville Goddard, 2015)

HSPs and the Search for Meaning

Spirituality means many different things to different people. But from my clinical experience it might mean for many HSPs something like 'that which lies beyond the present point of achievement — that which leads to a higher goal — a fuller expression of life' (Fraser, 2019). Most HSPs need to find meaning and purpose in their everyday work and life — their 'present point of achievement' at any moment needs to lead 'to a higher goal.' Most need to take part in work, for instance, that they believe leads in some way to a greater good or has a real (altruistic) purpose. As discussed in the chapter on HSPs and work, it has to be meaningful to them. Meaning for me was found in helping people to resolve health and wellbeing issues, my own included, and so improve the quality of Our existence.

HSPs are very capable of scanning their external environment while simultaneously having good awareness of their inner feeling responses and this ability moves them to deepen their consciousness on many levels. Greater sensitivity brings a heightened response across the spectrum of pain to pleasure and this intensity of experience tends to rouse a lifelong search for meaning. Their strong reactions to common everyday occurrences will cause the highly sensitive person to ask, 'What the hell was that all about?' It is no surprise that many HSPs describe their rich experience of the world in spiritual terms.

Dr Elaine Aron (2010) points out that most HSPs have been concerned from an early age about the existence or otherwise of some higher power, and about other questions of existence and death and why there is so much suffering in the world. Their answers to these questions may vary greatly. However, as we have seen from Aron and Aron's (1997) research, they are all expressed with great passion:

> from a strong religious faith since childhood to experiences with ghosts and angels ... [to] vehement atheism, ... the arguments were cogent and [always]

went beyond the usual wondering why God lets good people suffer. (Aron, 2010, pg.26)

Highly sensitive people also never require much prompting when it comes to discussing such issues. Indeed, Elaine Aron (2010) describes how the subject would always come up spontaneously in interviews before she got to her question on Spirituality and Self-Help, which she had placed last on her client interview protocol. My experience in my naturopathy practice has been the same. I must confess though, being an HSP myself, it only takes a hint of interest from a client and I'm happy to allow such a discussion to open up. My training permits me to call myself an 'Existentialist' if I find myself indulging too much!

For many HSPs, an awareness of suffering in the world and empathy for the pain of others is a product of their own experience of pain. Empathy is the extension of sensitivity to pain beyond the self to encompass the compassionate recognition of others' suffering and the desire to alleviate it. In the broader context of the world around us, we gain a sense of proportion about our own affairs and this often propels sensitive people into dedicating themselves to serving the needs of humanity in some way: 'Only the pure in heart can hear, only the gentle can respond' (*The Listening Pilgrim*).

The Wounded Healer

Carl Jung's description of what he termed the 'wounded healer' is very valid when considering HSPs' *empathic* worldview and their common choices to do work that helps others but heals themselves also. Their rich inner life lifts them to some great and exhilarating heights but it also takes them to many 'shadowy' and dark spaces in their mind. As Carl Jung put it: 'Knowing your own darkness is the best method for dealing with the darknesses of other people.'

We know HSPs generally put much time and energy into understanding deeper aspects of themselves — or anything else for that matter! I have seen in practice how this also applies to their approach to their health. As a natural therapist, I find my highly sensitive clients very receptive to taking a broader, more holistic and 'time-lined' vision of their health issues. They have a strong desire to understand the patterns and underlying (deeper) causes of their illness. If they can find meaning in their illness, tragedy or 'woundedness,' and discover the reasons and lessons to be learnt from their health crisis, it is then transformed into a 'healing' crisis. Enlightened and informed by the experience, they can put into practice behaviours and strategies to enable better ongoing health and wellbeing. In her book *Chiron and the Healing Journey* (2009) Melanie Reinhart states:

'suffering is present in everyone's life, but relating with wisdom and compassion to our own experience turns "poison into medicine."'

The strengths and weaknesses of our bodies and minds provide freedoms and limitations that help us to experience appropriate life lessons and personal growth. Life's struggle involves learning to live with one's unique and individual vulnerabilities, such as high sensitivity. Life's reward is discovering the profound qualities of the transpersonal Self that transcends individuality and connects to a world beyond conventional space and time. Perhaps the HSPs' at times fragile personal boundaries also make them more conscious of their intimate relationship with all other life forms. They can gain strength from their awareness that there is no such thing as splendid isolation; there is no separation between the various forms of life, for all are interdependent and all create one harmonious whole.

From ancient times to the present, the struggle with the limitations and incapacitating effects of our cumbersome physicality has driven the spirit to achieve greater refinement. This is how we grow as individuals. The physical body's boundaries are there to be exceeded by a developing mind that continually broadens its horizons. Ken Wilber's book *No Boundary: Eastern and Western Approaches to Personal Growth* (2001) expresses the belief that we are here to experience the ultimate metaphysical secret — that there are no boundaries in the universe. Boundaries are only illusions, products of the way we try to map and edit our reality. They may help us to get a sense of our own territory but reality is not so confined. All such boundaries and personal territories are permeable, and HSPs are reminded of this every day!

BIBLIOGRAPHY

Acevedo, B., Aron, E., Pospos, S., & Jessen, D. (2018). The functional highly sensitive brain: a review of the brain circuits underlying sensory processing sensitivity and seemingly related disorders. *Philos Trans R Soc Lond B Biol Sci., 373*(1744). doi:10.1098/rstb.2017.0161

Aron, A., Aron, E., Gabrieli, J., Hedden, T., Ketay, S. & Markus, H. (2010). Temperament trait of sensory processing sensitivity moderates cultural differences in neural response. *Social Cognitive and Affective Neuroscience.* doi: 10.1093/scan/nsq028

Aron, E. (2001). *The Highly Sensitive Person: how to thrive when the world overwhelms you.* Three Rivers Press: New York.

Aron, E. (2010). *Psychotherapy and the Highly Sensitive Person — improving outcomes for that minority of people who are the majority of clients.* Routledge: New York.

Aron, E. (2015). *The Highly Sensitive Child*. Thorsons: London.

Aron, E. Website: www.hsperson.com, https://hsperson.com/faq/hs-or-anxiety/

Aron, E., & Aron, A. (1997). Sensory-processing sensitivity and its relation to introversion and emotionality. *Journal of Personality and Social Psychology, 73*, 345-368.

Belsky, J. (2005). Differential susceptibility to rearing influence: An evolutionary hypothesis and some evidence. In B. Ellis & D. Bjorklund (Eds.), *Origins of the social mind: Evolutionary psychology and child development* (pp. 139–163). New York: Guilford.

Belsky, J., Bakermans-Kranenburg, M., & van IJzendoorn, M. (2007). For better and for worse: Differential Susceptibility to environmental influences. *Current Directions in Psychological Science, 16*(6), 300-304.

Berto, R. (2005). Exposure to restorative environments helps restore attentional capacity. *Journal of Environmental Psychology, 25*(3), 249-259. doi: 10.1016/j.jenvp.2005.07.001

Boyce, Thomas (2019) *The Orchid and the Dandelion: Why Some Children Struggle and How All Can Thrive*. Pan Macmillan: London.

Boyce, W. T., & Ellis, B. J. (2005). Biological sensitivity to context: I. An evolutionary-developmental theory of the origins and functions of stress reactivity. *Development and Psychopathology*, 17(2), 271-301.

Camoirano, A. (2017). Mentalizing makes parenting work: A review about parental reflective functioning and clinical interventions to improve it. *Frontiers of Psychology*, **8**, 14.

Davies, M., Stankov, L., & Roberts, R. (1998). Emotional intelligence: In search of an elusive construct. *Journal of Personality and Social Psychology, 75*, 989-1015.

Dimitroff, S., Kardan, O., Necka, E., Decety, J., Berman, M., & Norman, G. (2017) Physiological dynamics of stress contagion. *Scientific Reports* 7: 6168.
doi: 10.1038/s41598-017-05811-1

Ellis, B. and D. Bjorklund (Eds.), *Origins of the social mind: Evolutionary psychology and child development* (pp. 139–163). New York: Guilford.

Fraser, D. (2019). *Festival of Aquarius*. Lucis Trust: London.

Frijda, N., Kuipers, P., & Ter Schure, E. (1989). Relations among emotion, appraisal, and emotional action readiness. *Journal of Personality and Social Psychology, 57*, 212-228.

Glenberg, A. (2011). Monkey See, Monkey Do? The Role of Mirror Neurons in Human Behavior. *Association for Psychological Science*. www.psychologicalscience.org/news/releases/monkey-see-monkey-do-the-role-of-mirror-neurons-in-human-behavior

Goddard, Neville (2015). *The Complete Reader, Volume 1*. Watchmaker Publishing: Gearhart, Oregon.

Heller, L., LaPierre, A. (2012) *Healing Developmental Trauma: How Early Trauma Affects Self-Regulation, Self-Image, and the Capacity for Relationship*. North Atlantic Books: Berkeley, California.

Henderson-Wilson, Claire. (2008) *Healthy parks, healthy people — the health benefits of contact with nature in a park context*. Deakin University: Melbourne.

Hill, Maria, from Sensitive Evolution. Website: www.sensitiveevolution.com

Jaeger, B. (2004). *Making Work Work for the Highly Sensitive Person*. McGraw-Hill: New York.

Jung, C.G. (1955) Vesuch Einer Darstellung Der Psychanalytischen Theorie. Zuric: Rascher & Cie (First published in 1913.)

Jung, C.G. (1976) *Psychological Types*. Princeton, NJ: Princeton University Press.

Kaplan, S. (1995) The restorative benefits of nature: Toward an integrative framework.
Journal of Environmental Psychology, 15:3, 169-182. doi:10.1016/0272-4944(95)90001-2

Kaminski, P., Katz, R. (Eds.) (1994). *Flower Essence Repertory — A comprehensive guide to North American and English flower essences for emotional and spiritual well-being*. The Flower Essence Society: Nevada City. Website: www.fesflowers.com

Kogan, J. 2004 *The Long Shadow of Temperament*. Belknap Press Harvard University Press: London.

Kuo, F. & Sullivan, W. (2001) Environment and Crime in the Inner City: Does Vegetation Reduce Crime? *Environment and Behaviour*, 33: 3, 343-367. doi:10.1177/0013916501333002

Lombard, A. (2014). *Sensory Intelligence — why it matters more than IQ and EQ.* Metz Press: Welgemoed, South Africa. Website: www.sensoryintelligence.com

Lo, I. (2018). *Emotional Sensitivity and Intensity — how to manage emotions as a sensitive person.* Holder & Stroughton: London.

McGilchrist, I. (2012). *The Master and His Emissary — the divided brain and the making of the western world.* Yale University Press: London.

McKinnon, P. (2011) *Living Calm in a Busy World.* David Lovell Publishing: Melbourne.

Masuda, T. & Nisbett, R. (2001). Attending holistically vs. analytically: Comparing the context sensitivity of Japanese and Americans. *Journal of Personality and Social Psychology*, 81, 922-934. doi: 10.1037/0022-3514.81.5.922

Meares, A. (1970). *Relief Without Drugs — how to conquer tension, pain and anxiety.* Fontana Books: Sydney

Meares, A., (1987). *Life Without Stress — the self-management of stress.* Greenhouse Publications: Melbourne.

Mesich, K. (2001) *The Sensitive Person's Survival Guide — an alternative health answer to emotional sensitivity and depression.* Ansuz Press: Minneapolis, MN.

Moore, T. (1992) *Care of the Soul — a guide for cultivating depth and sacredness in everyday life.* HarperCollins: New York.

Nerenberg, J. (2021) *Divergent Mind — thriving in a world that wasn't designed for you.* Harper One: San Francisco.
O'Loughlin, Kelly. Website: www.highlysensitiveperson.net

Orloff, J. (2018) *Empath's Survival Guide: Life Strategies for Sensitive People.* Sounds True: Boulder, Colorado.

Ostaseski, F. (2017) *The Five Invitations — discovering what death can teach us about living fully.* Flatiron Books: New York.

Positive Psychology Program B.V. (2019). Gandhiplein 16 6229HN Maastricht, The Netherlands. Website: www.positivepsychologyprogram.com

Reichart, M. (2019) *How to Raise a Boy: The Power of Connection to Build Good Men* TarcherPerigee: New York.

Reinhart, Melanie (2009) *Chiron and the Healing Journey.* Starwalker Press: London.

Rosenberg, M.B. (2003). *Nonviolent communication: A language of Life.* Puddledancer Press: Encinitas, California.

Russell, Melissa (2017). *Why Highly Sensitive People Need Minimalism.* www.simplelionheartlife.com/highly-sensitive-people-need-minimalism/

Sand, I. (2016) *Highly Sensitive People in an Insensitive World — how to create a happy life.* Jessica Kingsley: London.

Sand, I. (2018) *On Being an Introvert or Highly Sensitive Person — a guide to boundaries, joy and meaning.* Jessica Kingsley: London.

Sand, I. (2017) *Tools for Helpful Souls — especially for highly sensitive people who provide help either on a professional or private level.* Jessica Kingsley: London.

Schwartz, M. (2020) at Leading Edge Parenting. Website: www.leadingedgeparenting.com

Schwarz, N. (2012). Feelings-as-information theory. In P. A. M. Van Lange, A. W. Kruglanski, & E. T. Higgins (Eds.), *Handbook of theories of social psychology* (pp. 289-308). Sage Publications Ltd: Thousand Oaks, California.

Solo, A. (2019). *Do Highly Sensitive People Have Autism?* www.psychologytoday.com/us/blog/highly-sensitive-refuge/201905/do-highly-sensitive-people-have-autism

Tartakovsky, Margarita, *PsychCentral.com* 14 August, 2017. www.psychcentral.com/authors/margarita-tartakovsky-ms

Wells, M. (2015). *The Essential Flower Essence Book — flower essences for living, healing, personal growth and transformation.* Wells Naturopathic Centre: Melbourne

White, Diana, (2014). *7 Advantages of Being a Sensitive Person.* www.womanitely.com/advantages-being-sensitive-person/ Website: www.womanitely.com

Wiens, S., Mezzacappa, E. S., & Katkin, E. S. (2000). Heartbeat detection and the experience of emotions. *Cognition and Emotion, 14*(3), 417-427. doi: 10.1080/026999300378905

Wilber, Ken (2001). *No Boundary: Eastern and Western Approaches to Personal Growth.* Shambhala: Boston, Massachusetts

Zeff, T. (2010). *The Strong Sensitive Boy — help your son become a happy, confident man.* Prana Publishing: Oxenford, Queensland, Australia. Website: drtedzeff.com

Other books by Mark Wells

Emotion Healed & Harnessed: Create the Life You Desire with Flower Essence, Meditation & Emotion-Focused Therapies. Melbourne: HSP Health, 2025

The Essential Flower Essence Book: Flower Essences for Living, Healing, Personal Growth and Blossoming.
Melbourne: HSP Health, 2023.

Simon, A. & Wells, M. *The Cosmos in the Cauldron: Combining the Wisdom of Astrology and the Innate Intelligence of Plants and Minerals to Heal and Grow.*
Melbourne: Mark Wells, 2019.

Twelve Dynamic Elements of Good Health: The Tissue Salts.
Melbourne: Mark Wells, 2016.

The Bach Flowers Today. Melbourne: Mark Wells, 2013.

CONTACT

Mark Wells

Private Practice
HSP Health
PO Box 79
Kew, 3101
Melbourne, Australia.
Phone: 0409985970

Website: hsphealth.com.au

For all information about
Mark's media and private practice,
and about ordering his other books.

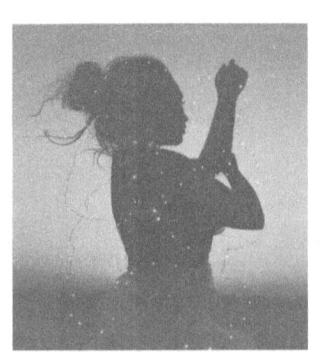

www.ingramcontent.com/pod-product-compliance
Lightning Source LLC
Chambersburg PA
CBHW031242290426
44109CB00012B/399